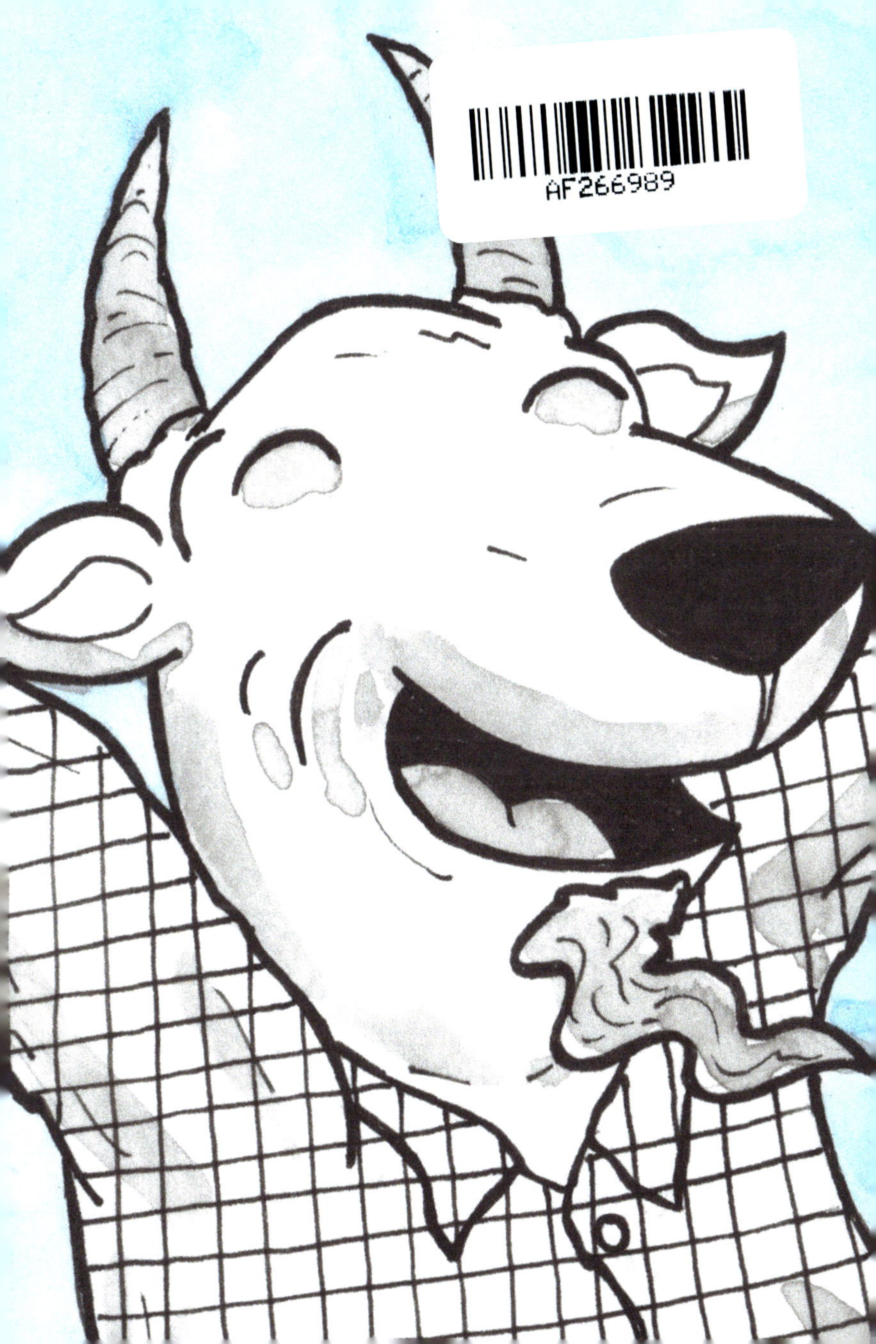

AF266989
AF266

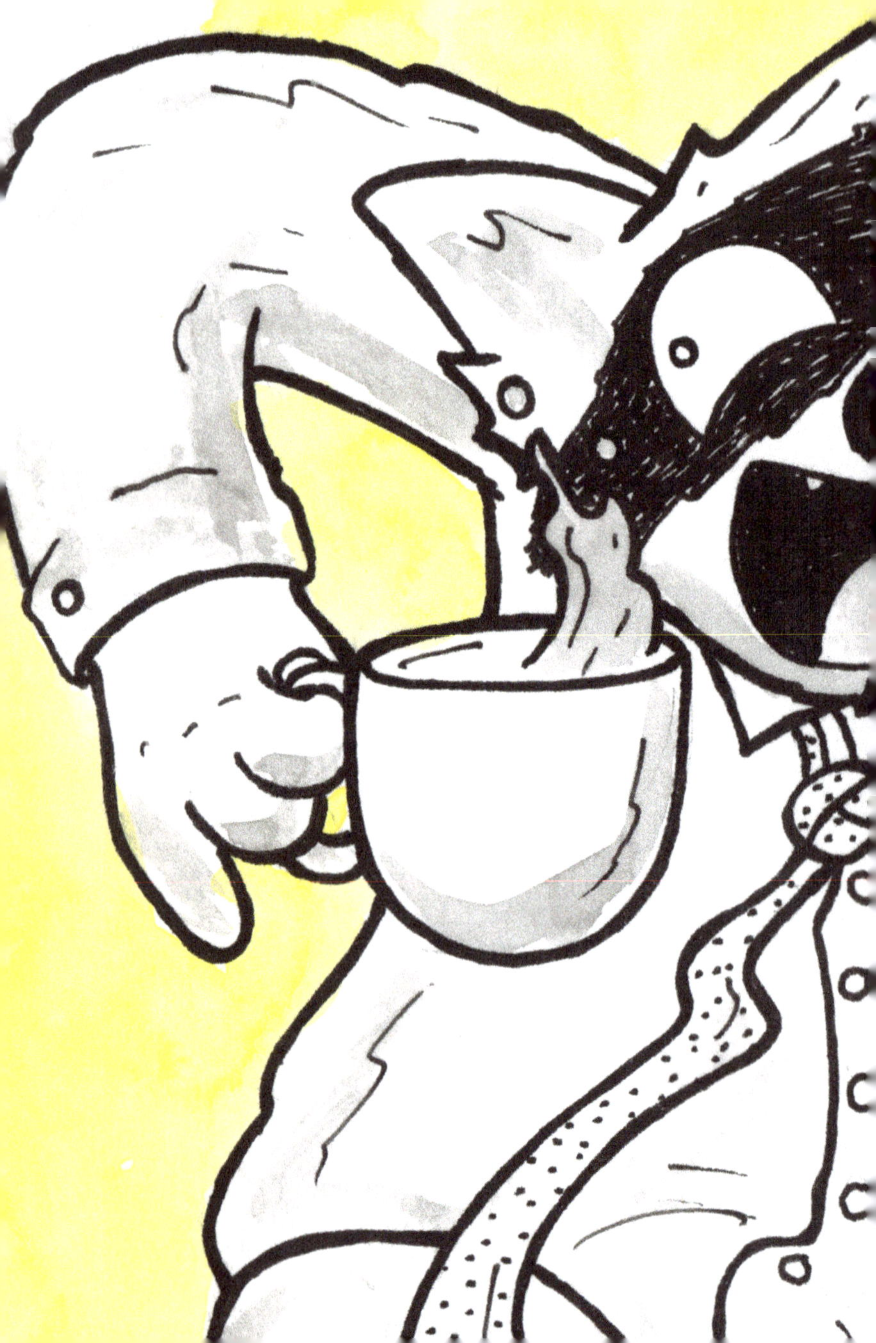

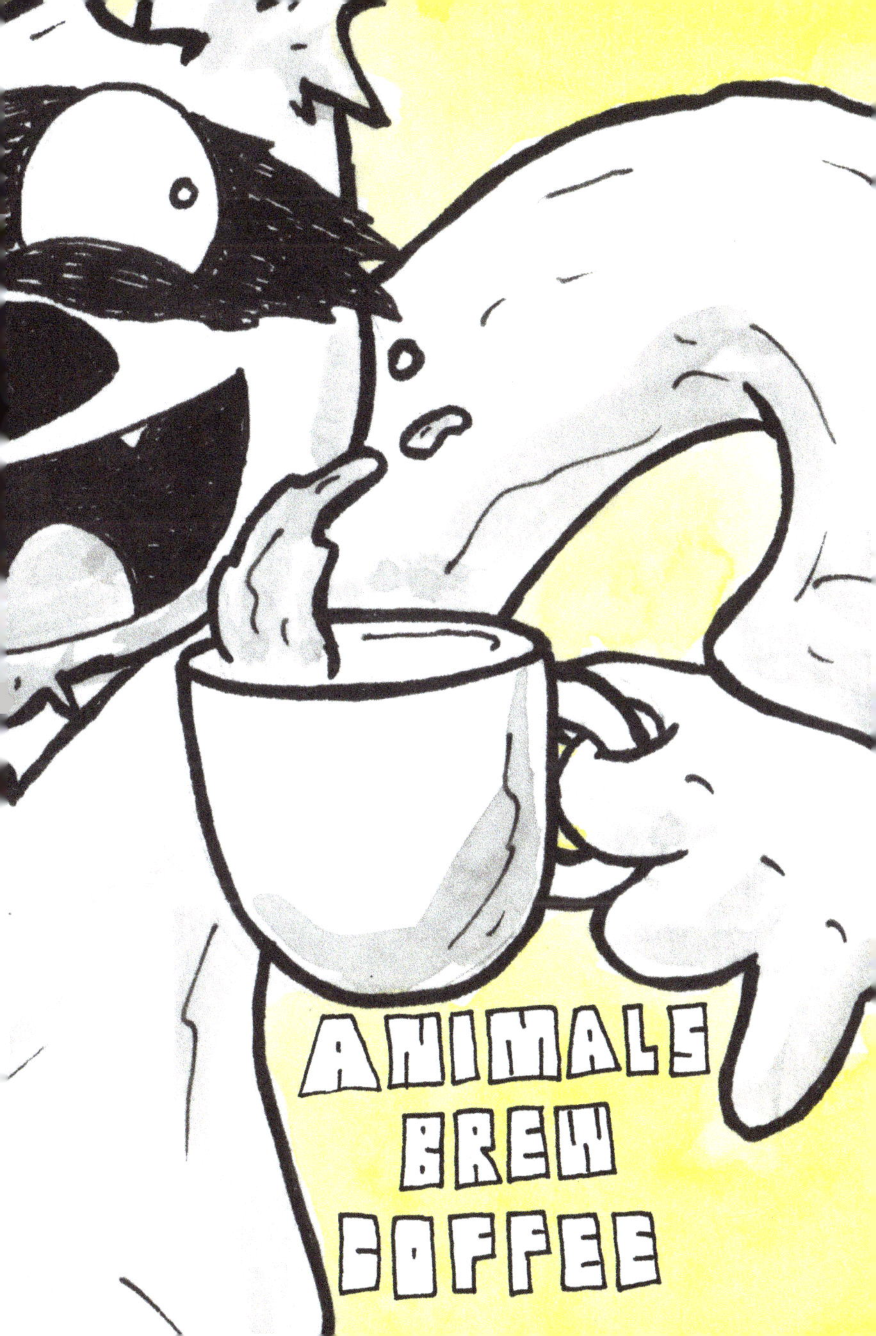

ANIMALS
BREW
COFFEE

ANIMALS BREW COFFEE © 2016
BY P. CALAVARA
PUBLISHED BY NEVER KNOWS BOOKS
ISBN- 978-0-9964120-1-8

ORIGINALLY PRESENTED ONE-PAGE-PER-DAY ON THE
WALLS OF BATDORF & BRONSON COFFEE SHOP IN OLYMPIA, WA
AS WELL AS ON MISTER INTERNET AT: RACCOONTEURS.COM.
WHEN NOT BICKERING WITH EACH OTHER ABOUT THE STATE
OF THE STUDIO COFFEE POT, P. CALAVARA CAN BE FOUND IN
BEAUTIFUL OLYMPIA, TRADING ROBOTS FOR LATTES.

*CALAVARA.COM *NEVERKNOWS.COM*

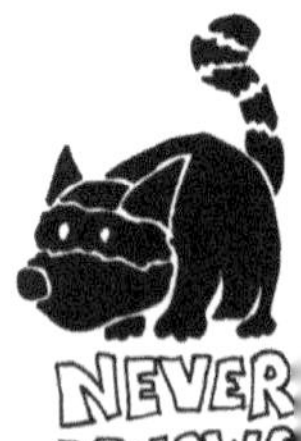

THIS BOOK IS FOR JENYA—
WHO STILL BOTHERS TO
ANSWER MY RANDOM
COFFEE QUESTIONS.

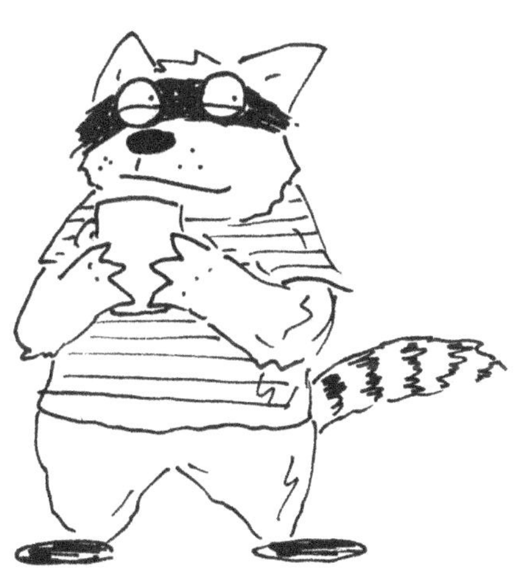

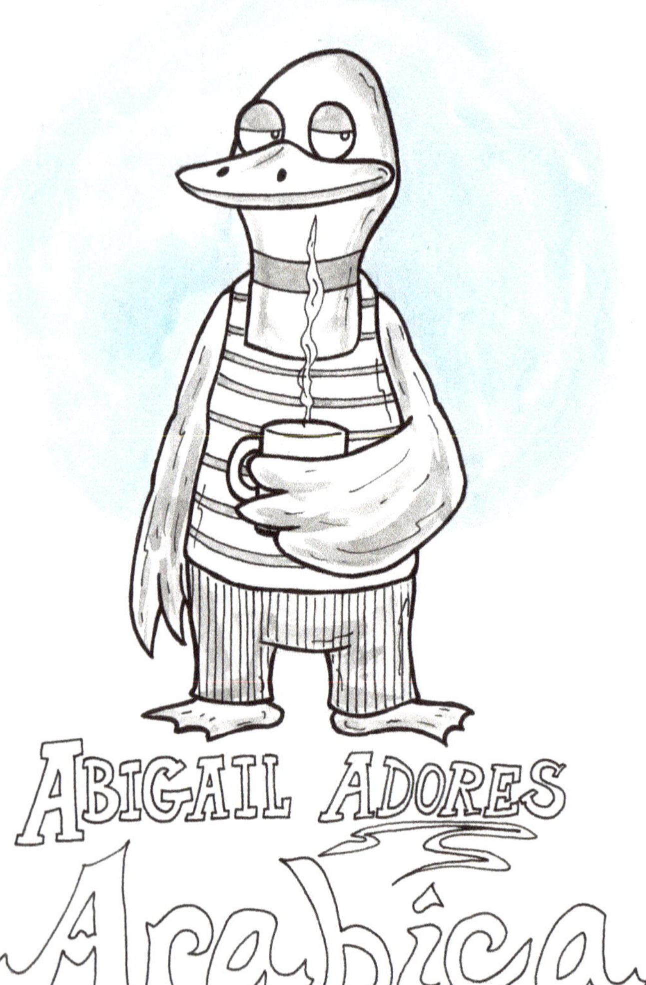
ABIGAIL ADORES
Arabica

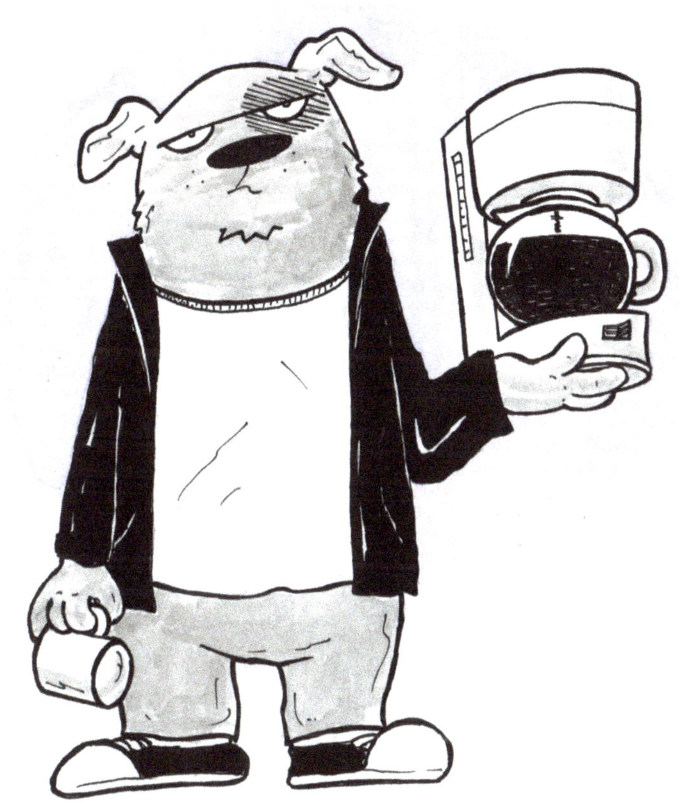

Bernard brews it
BLACK

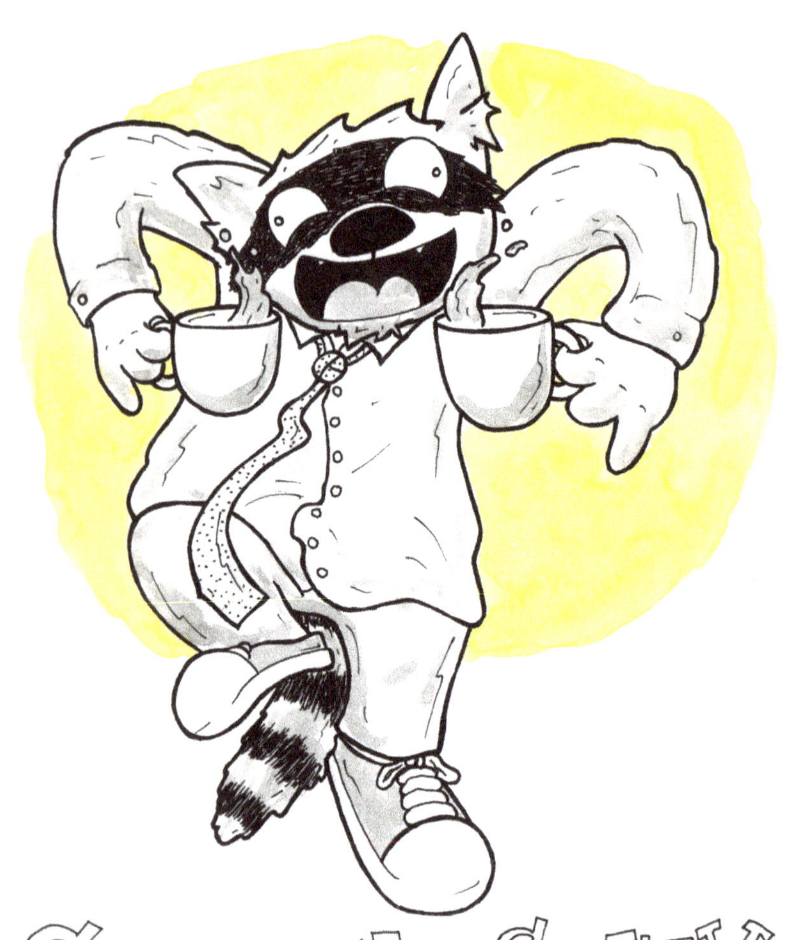
CAMDEN is CRAZY
For
Cappuccino

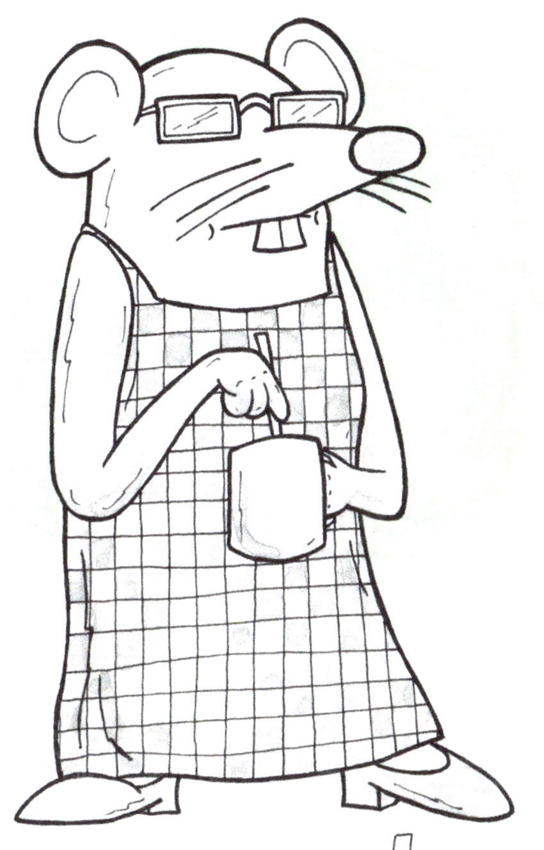

Desiree drinks
decaf drip daily

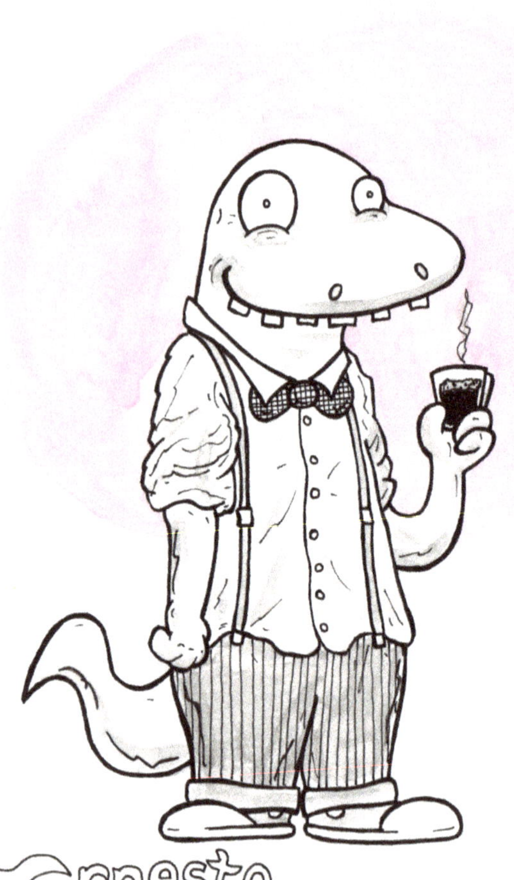

Ernesto is energized by Espresso

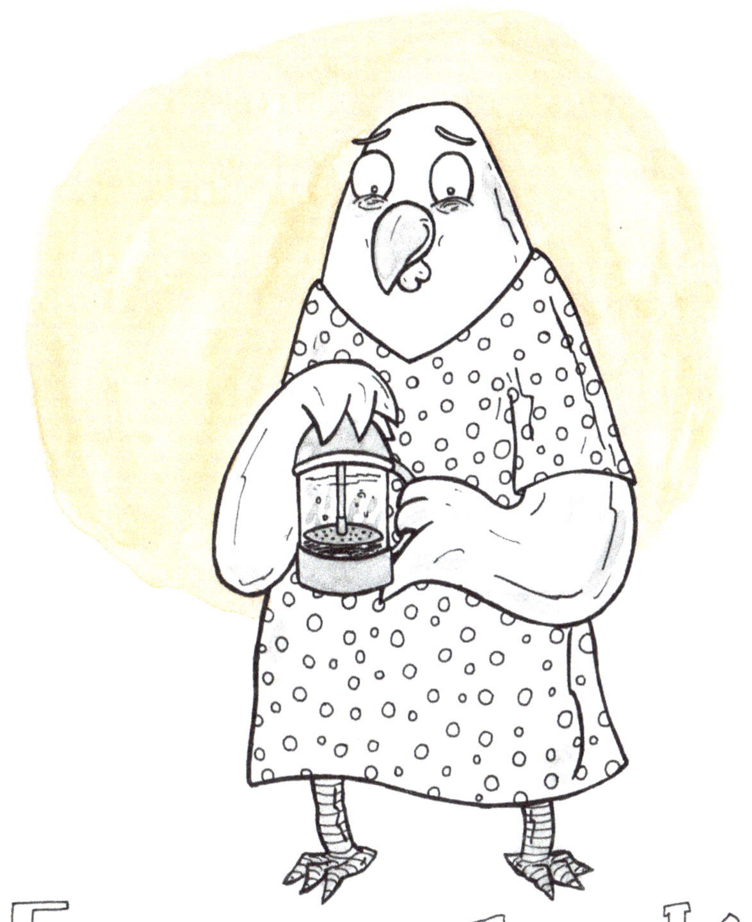

Francine is Frantic for French Press

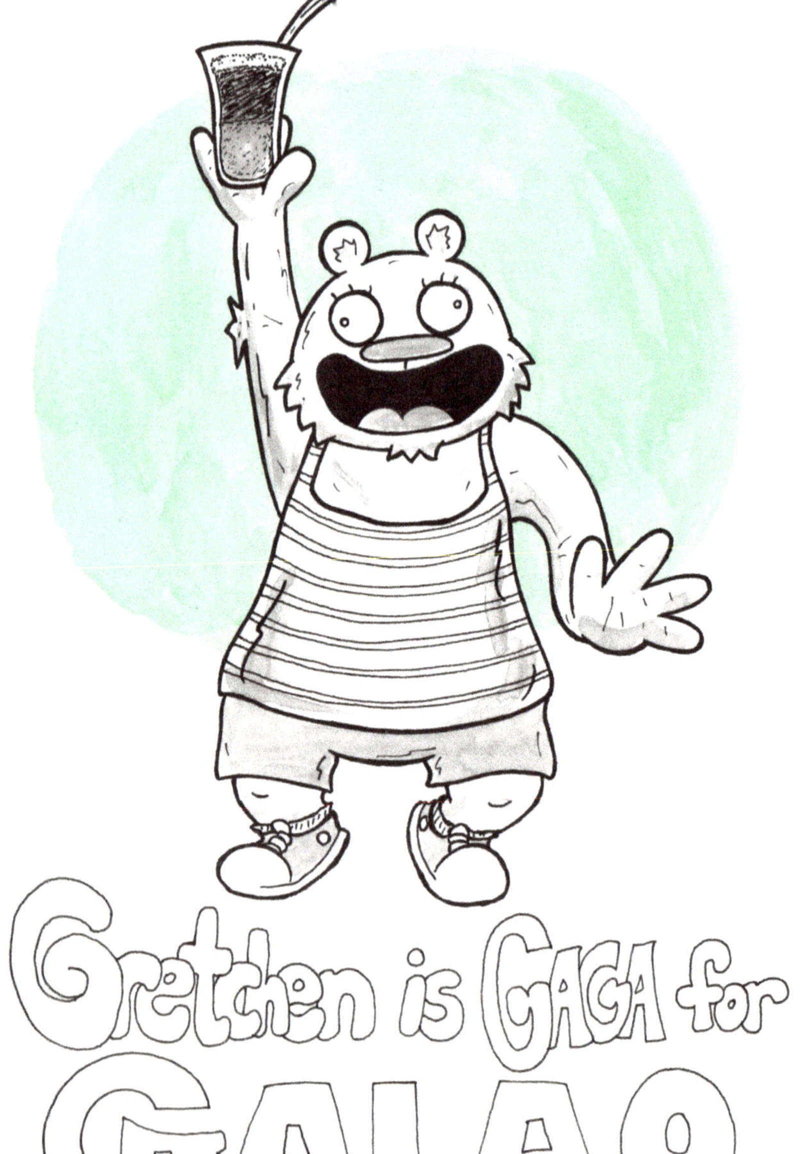

Gretchen is GAGA for
GALAO

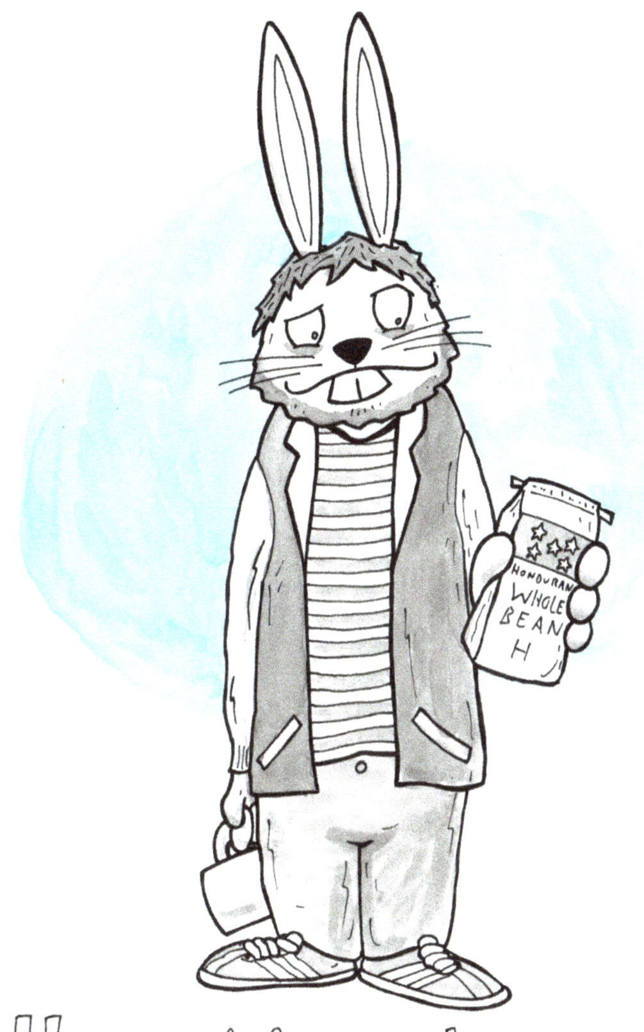

Harold has a hankerin' for

HONDURAN

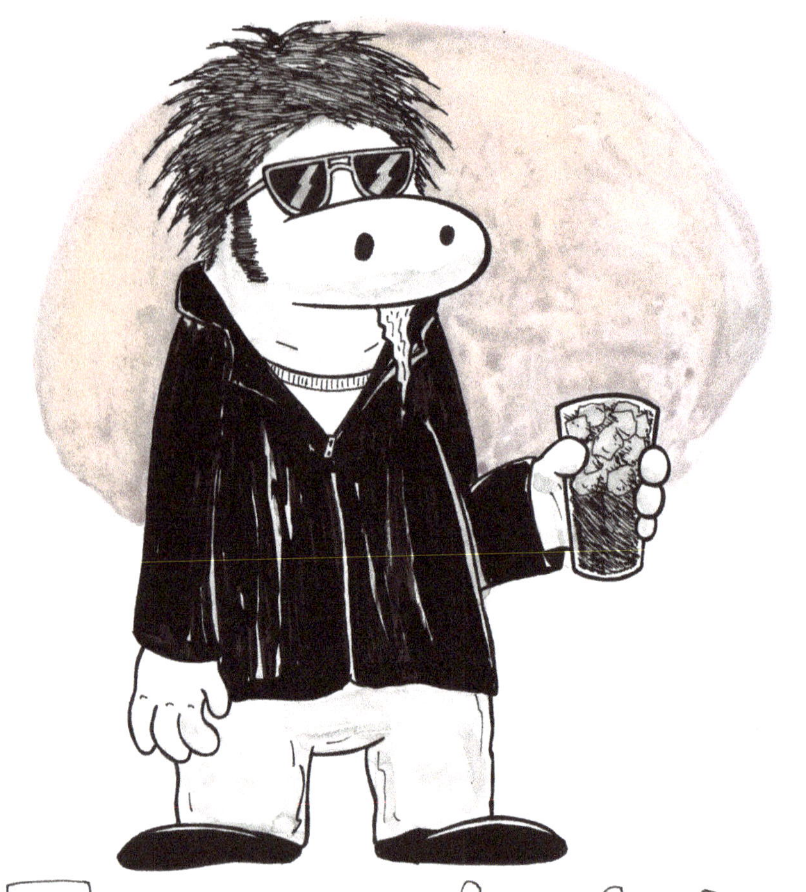

Isaac insists
-on-
ICED INSTANT

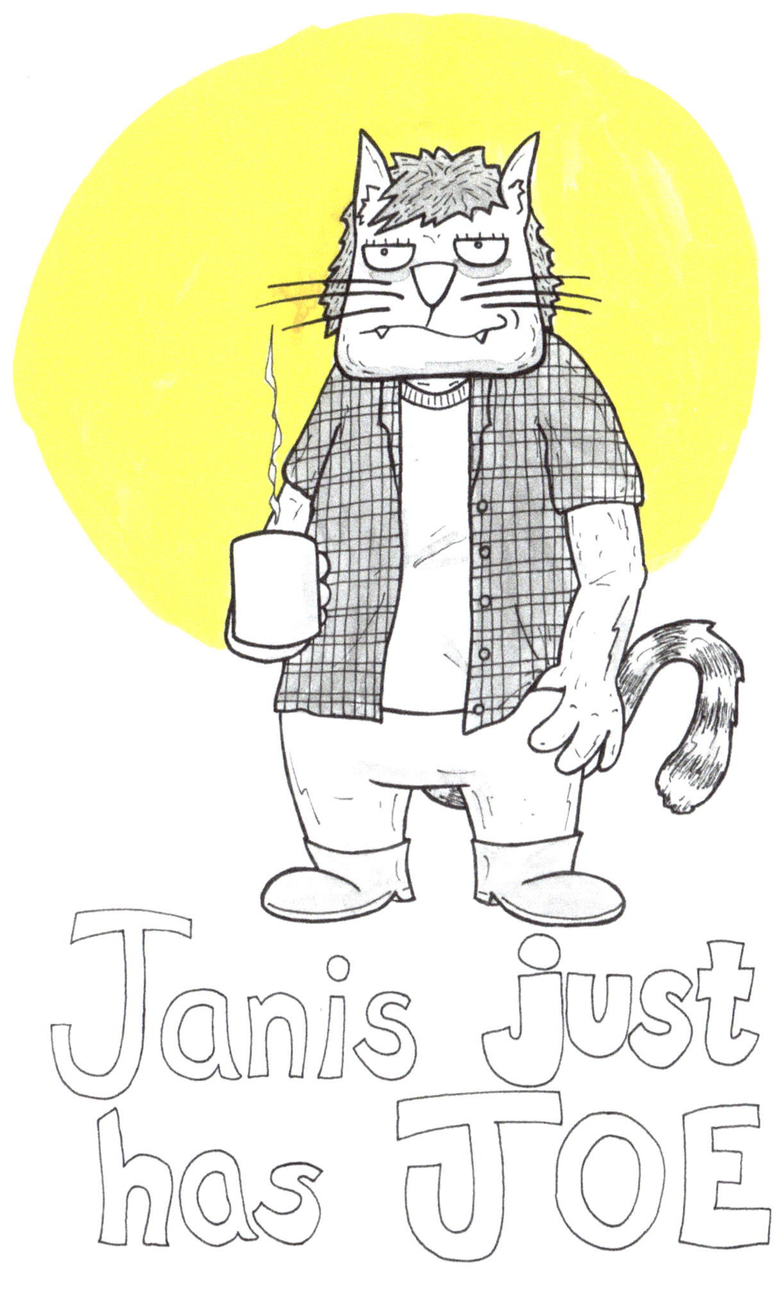
Janis just has JOE

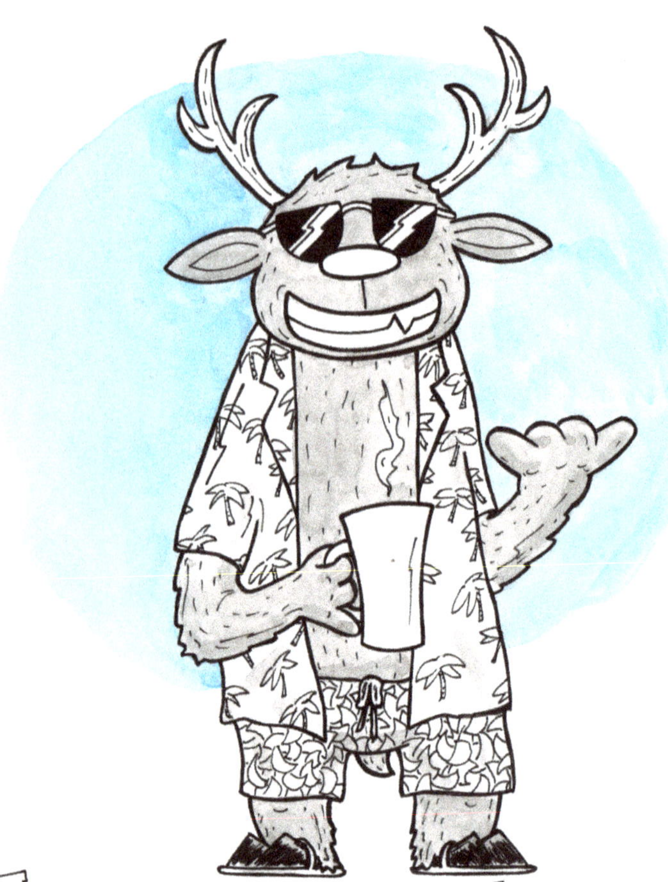

Kevin is Keen
on KONA

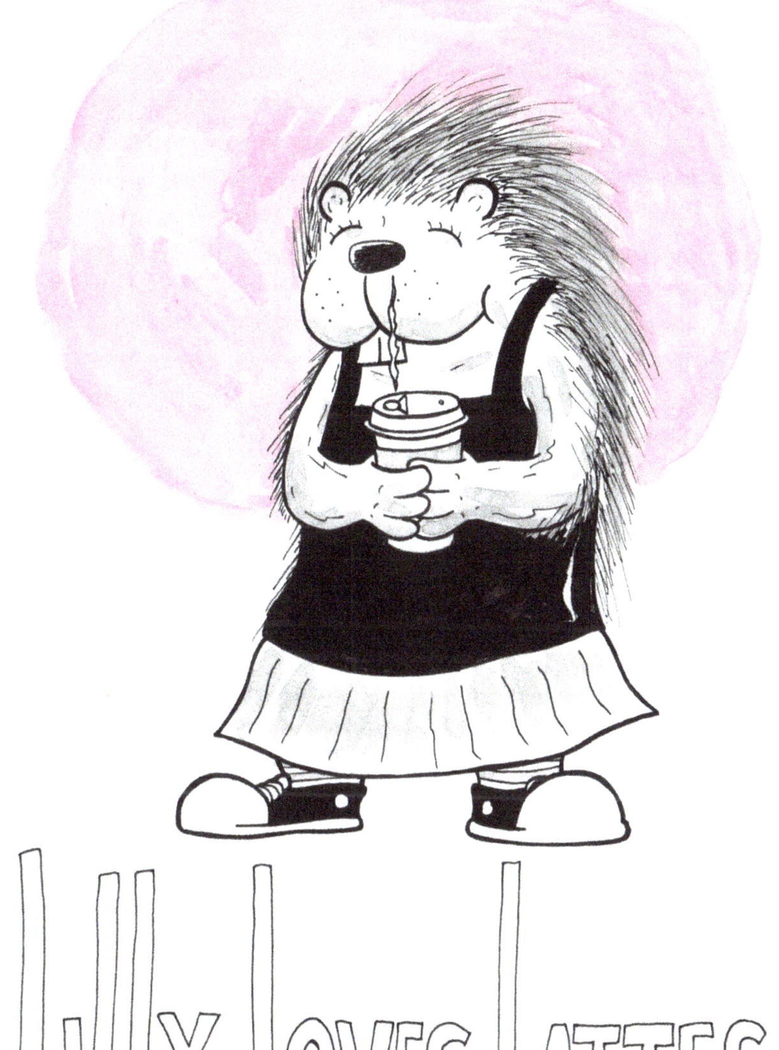

LiLLy Loves Lattes

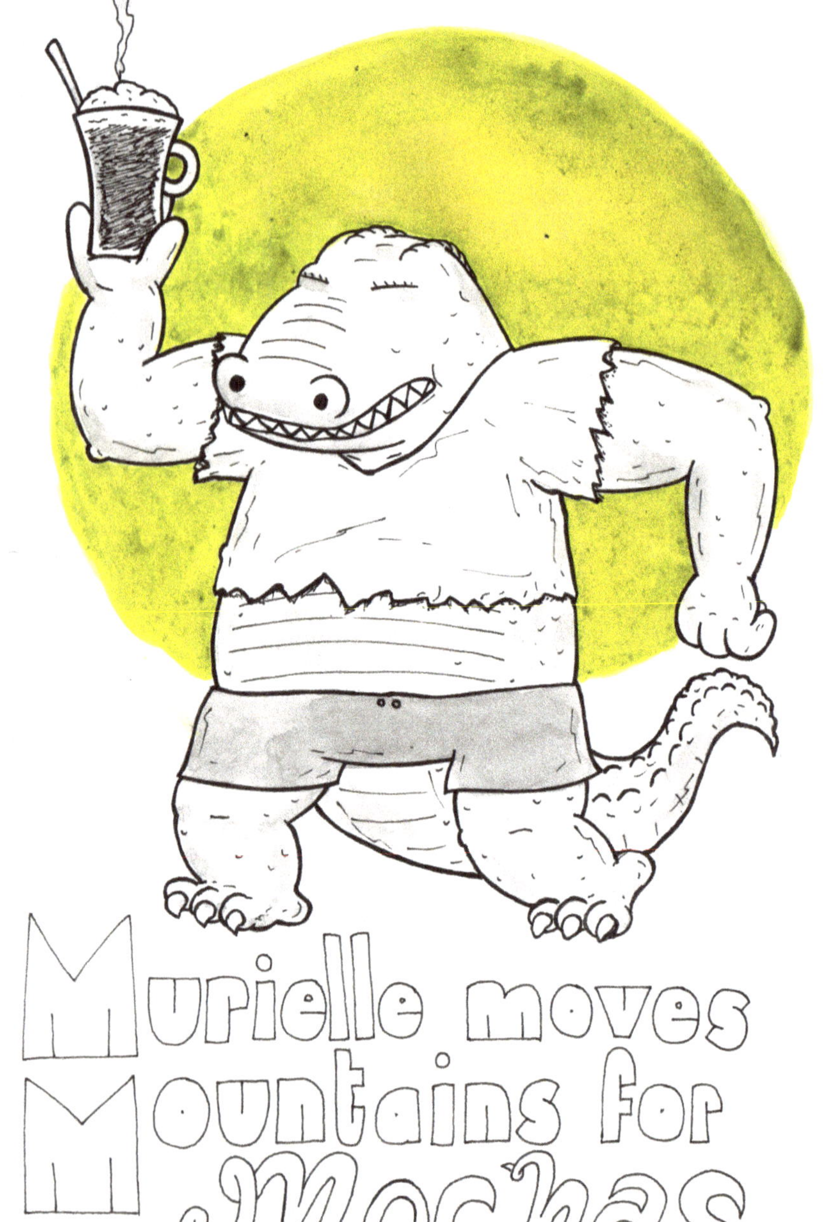
Murielle moves
Mountains for
Mochas

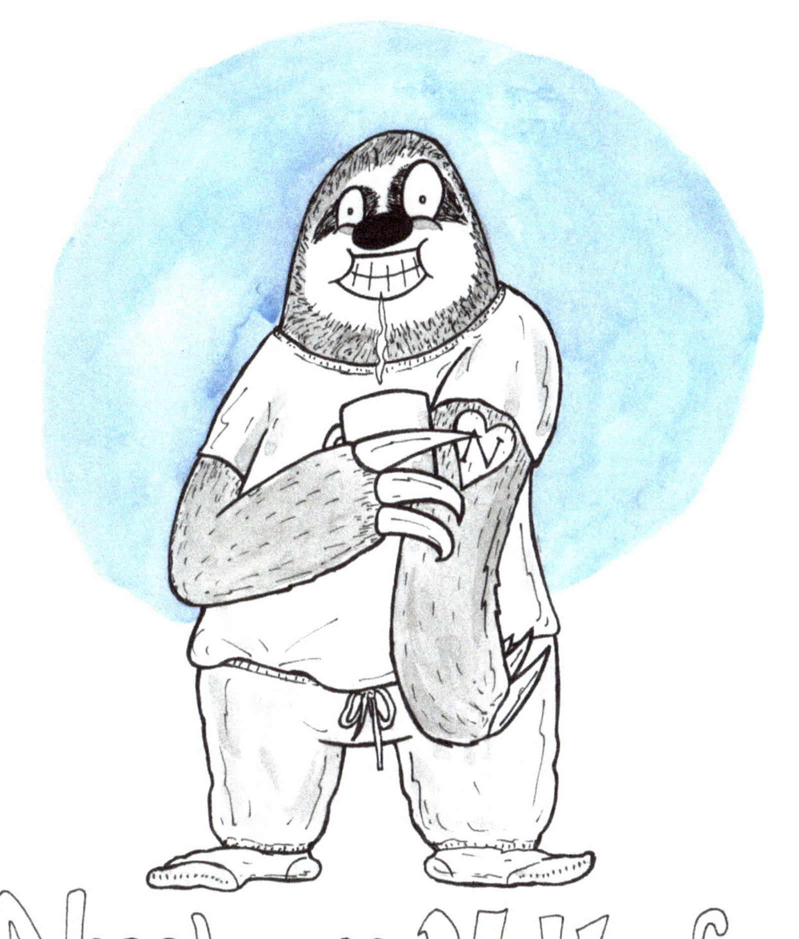

Nicolas is *Nutty* for the nicer notes of **NICARAGUAN**

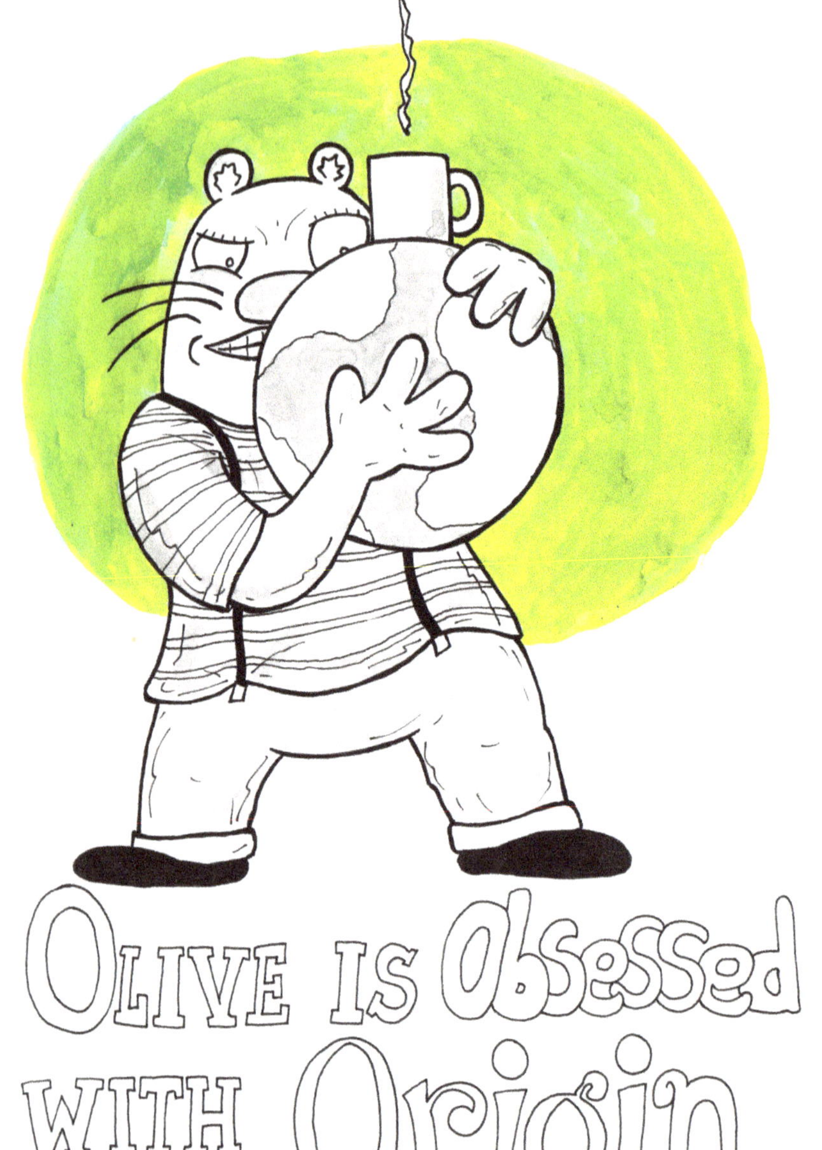

Olive is Obsessed with Origin

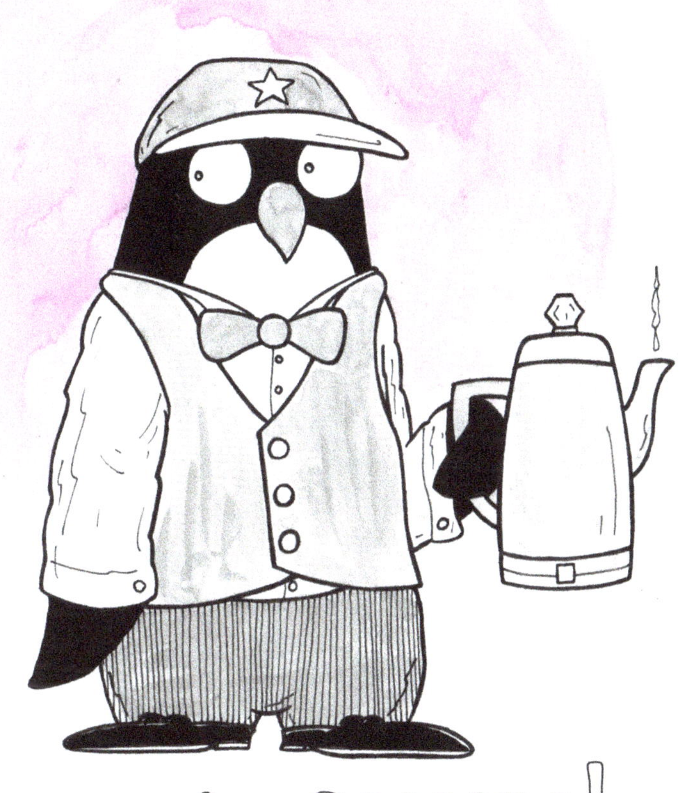

Pierre's personal preference is Probably for the Percolator

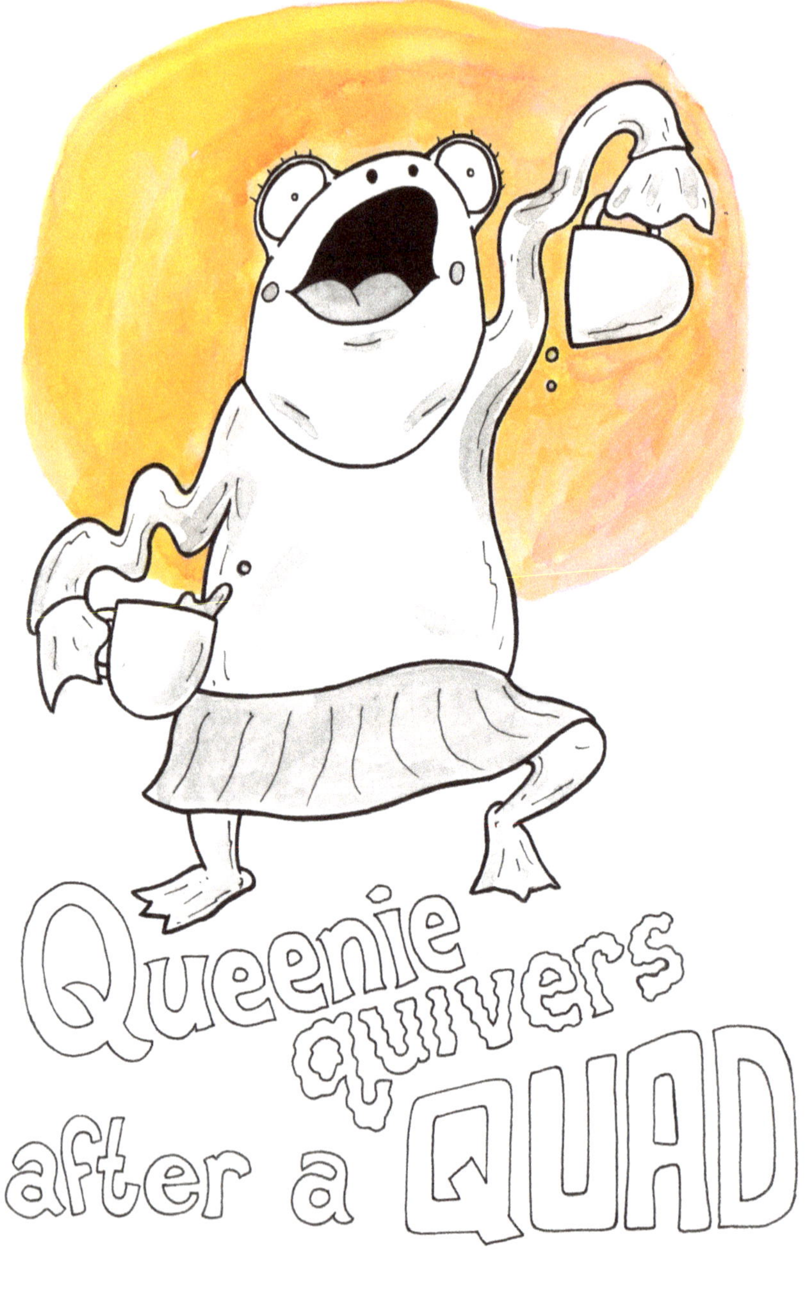
Queenie quivers after a QUAD

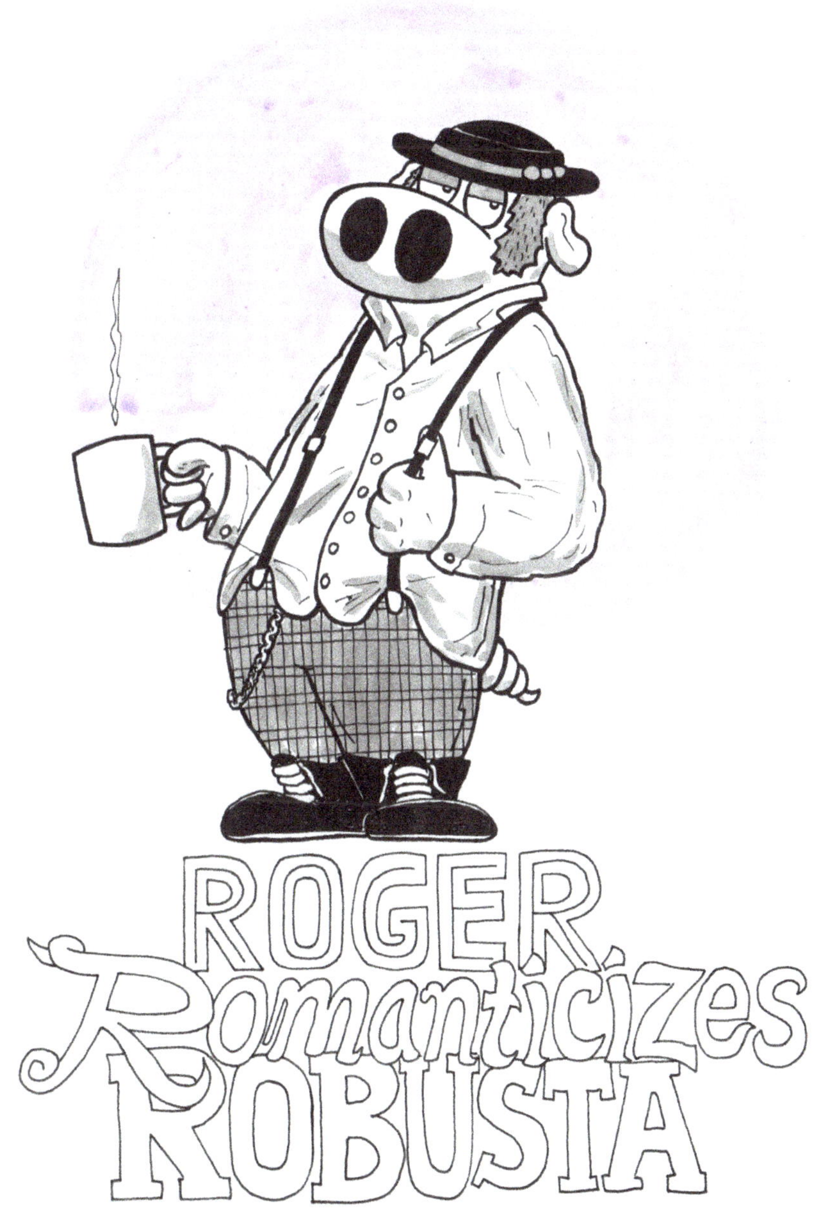

ROGER
Romanticizes
ROBUSTA

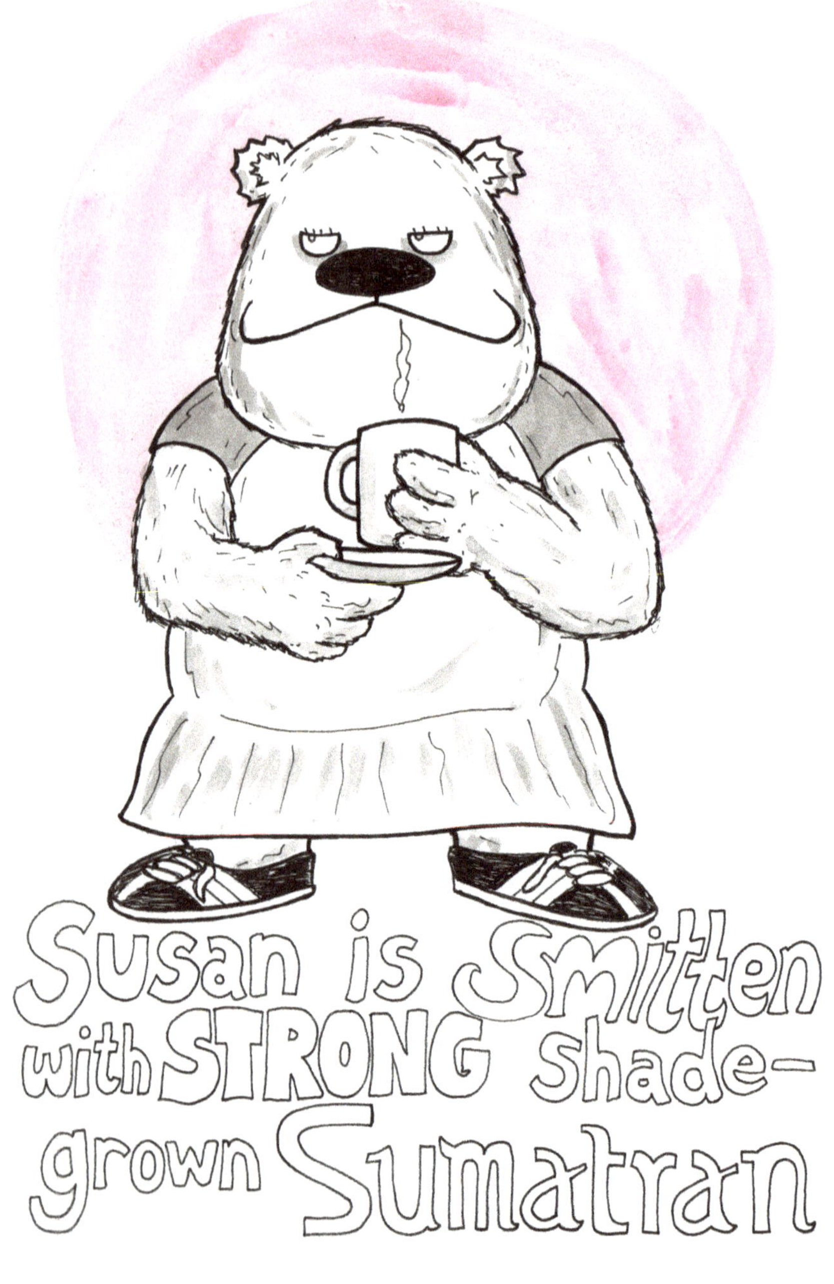

Susan is Smitten with STRONG shade-grown Sumatran

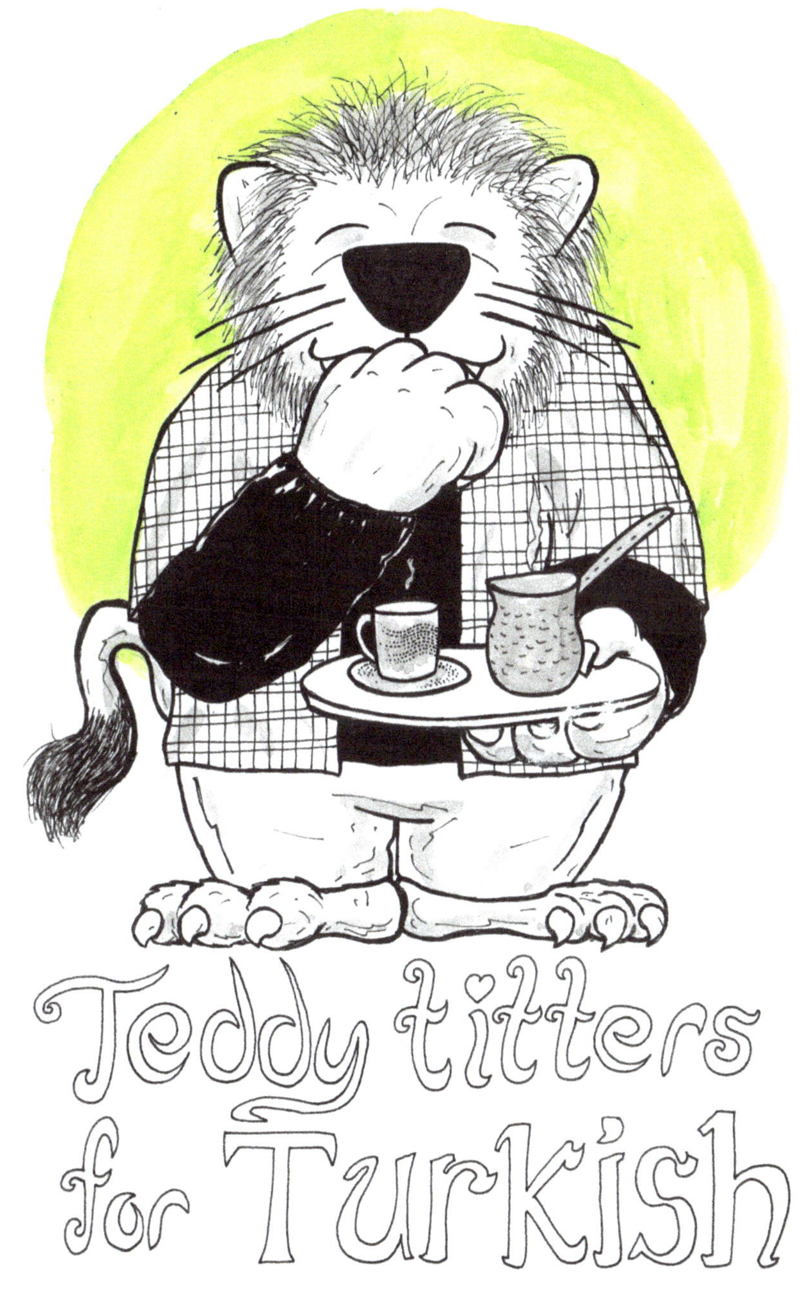
Teddy titters
for Turkish

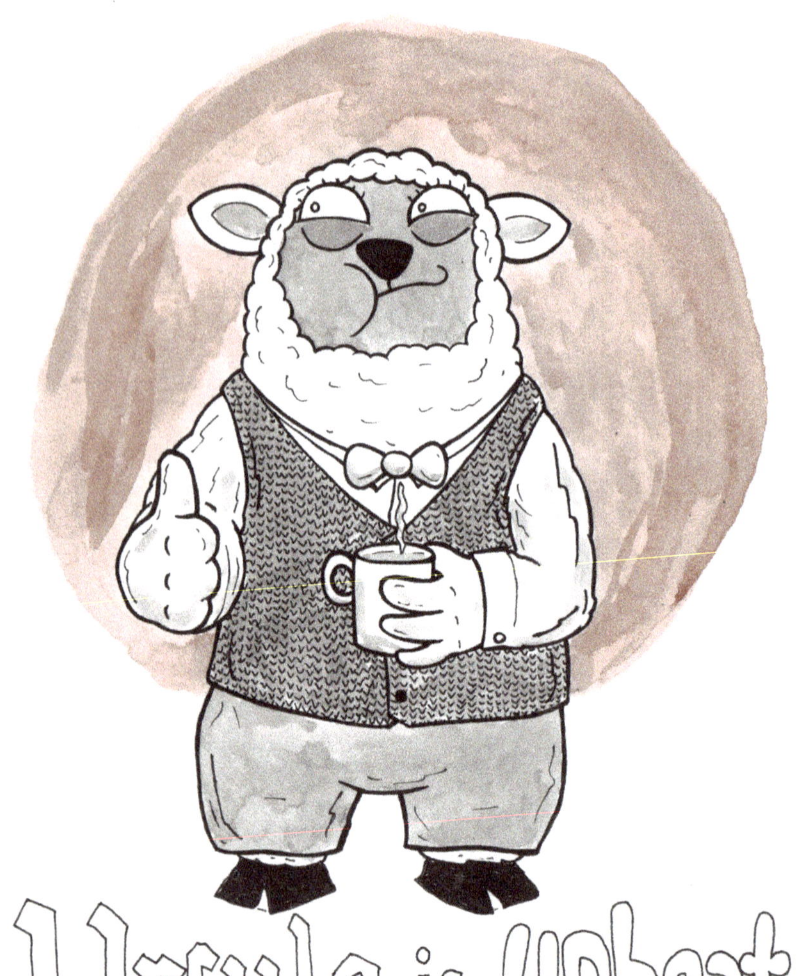

Ursula is Upbeat about UMAMI

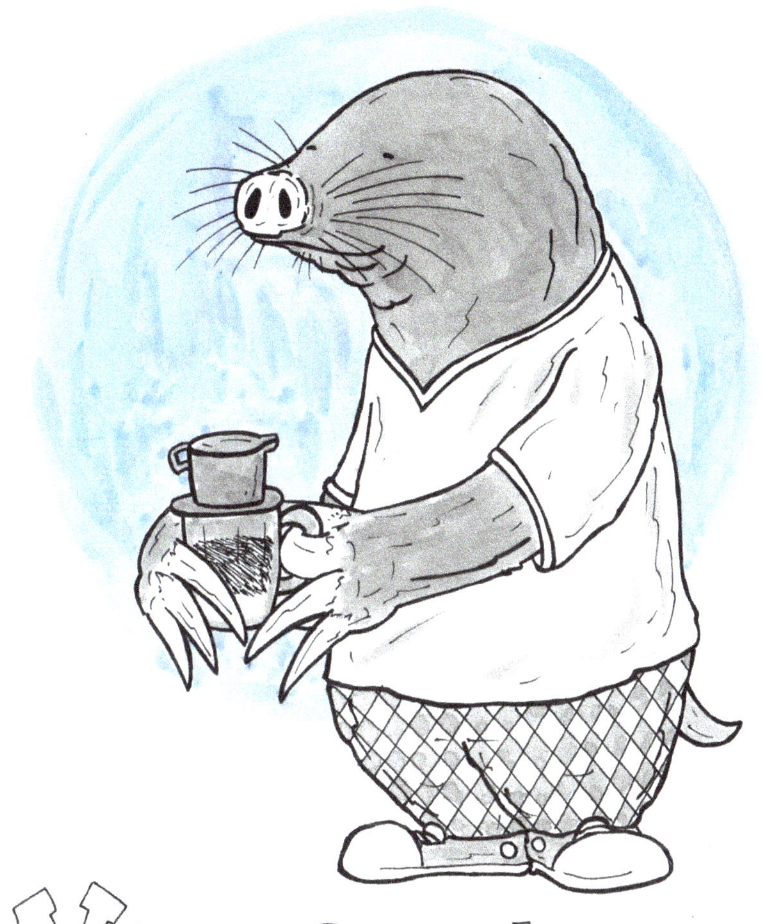

Vincent values
VIETNAMESE

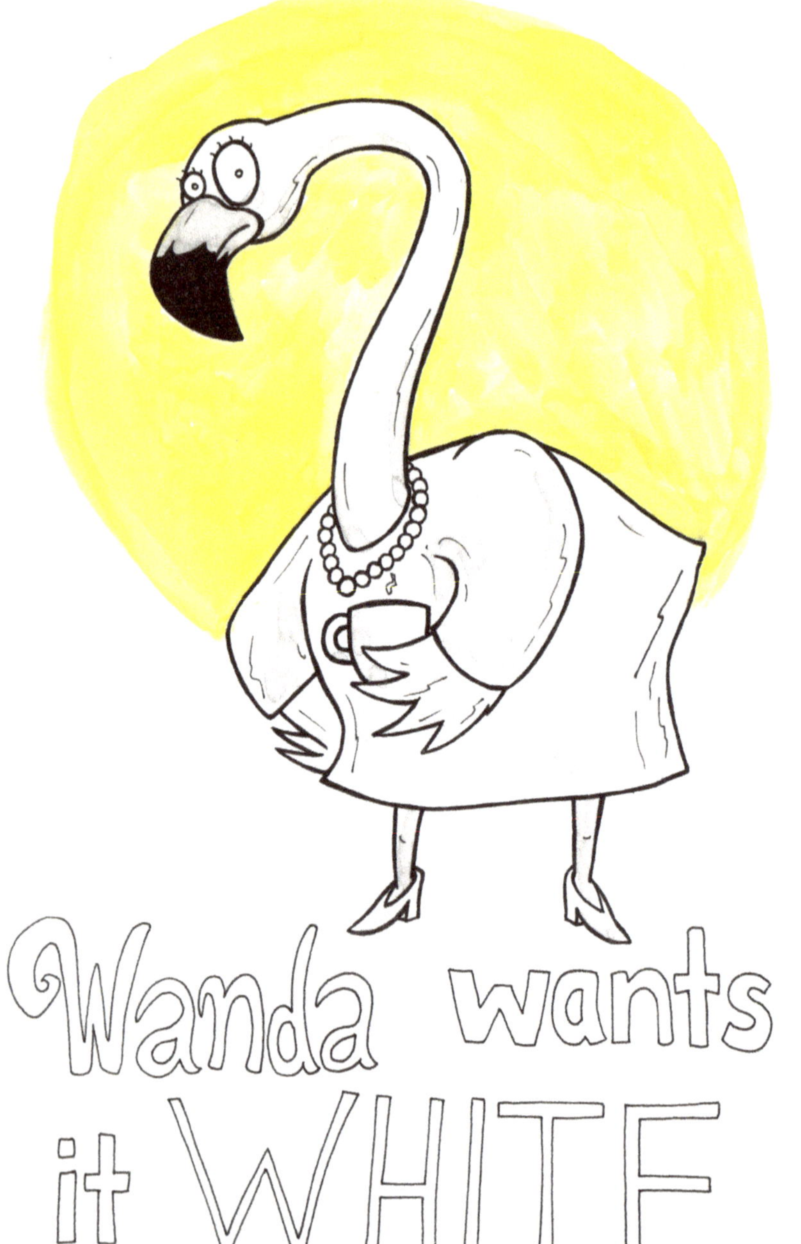

Wanda wants it WHITE

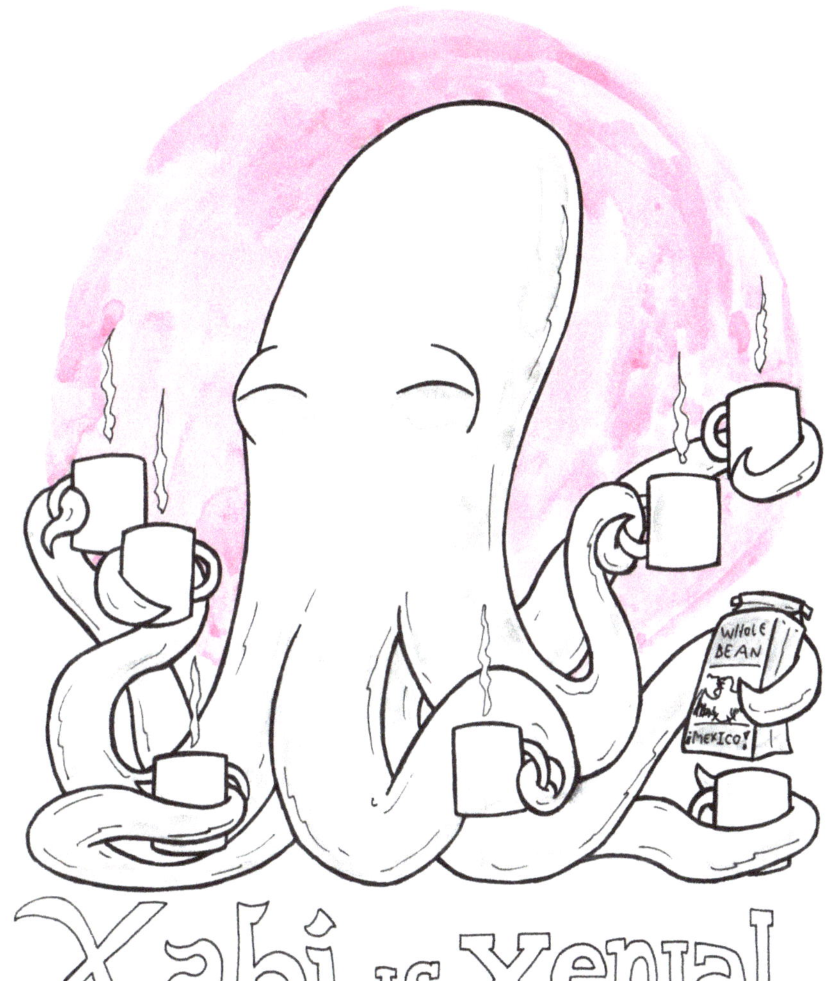

WHOLE BEAN
¡MEXICO!
Xabi is Xenial
with his XALAPAN

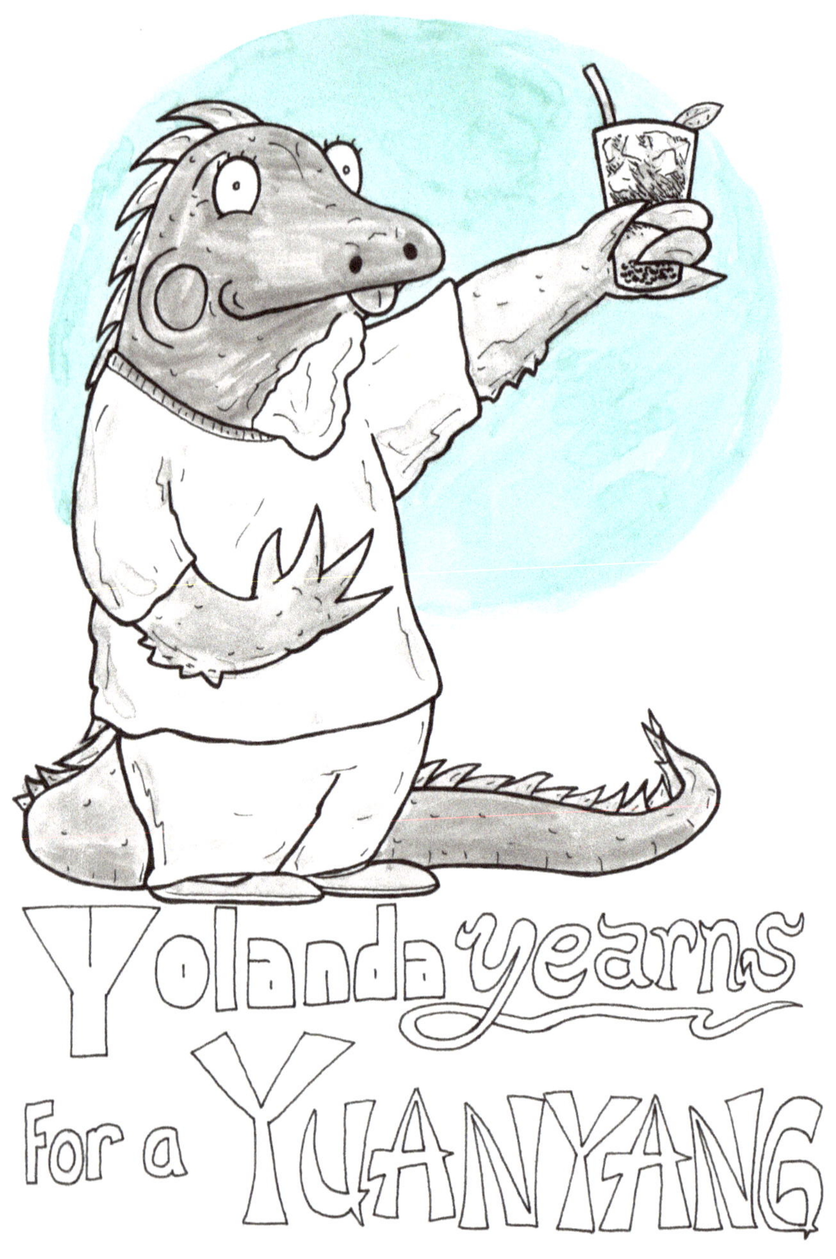

Yolanda yearns
for a YUANYANG

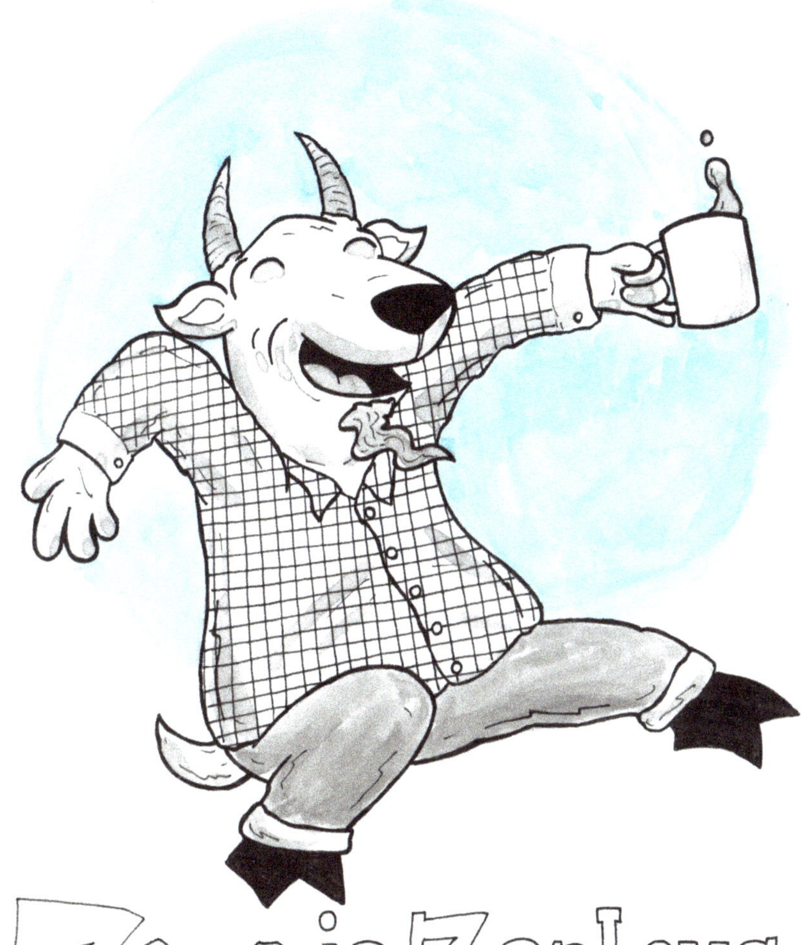

Zane is Zealous
about Zambian

Winter's Cruel Reign Flickers Beneath the Stern Gaze of Hot Drink

38 PAINTINGS AND 2 MORE PAINTINGS

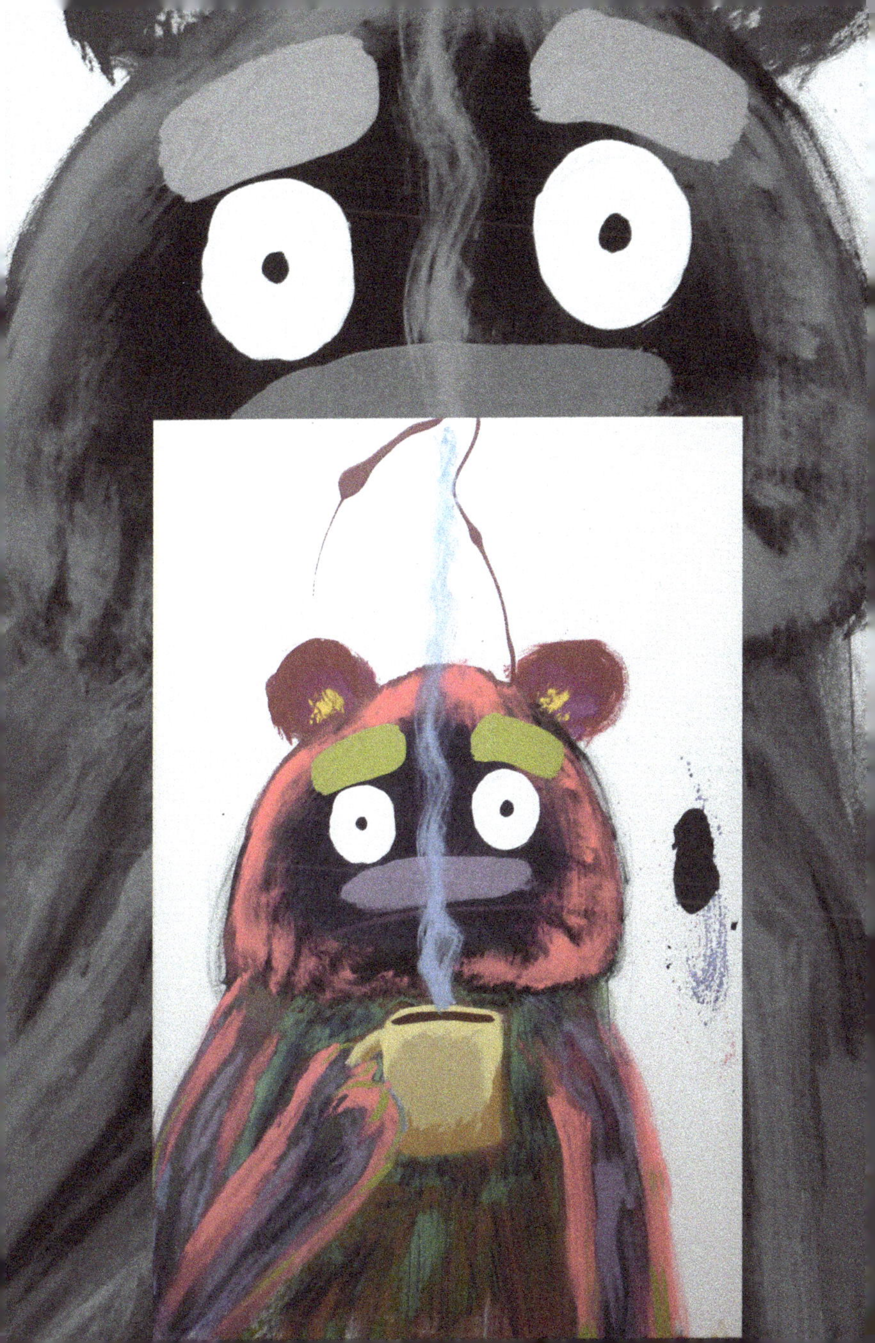

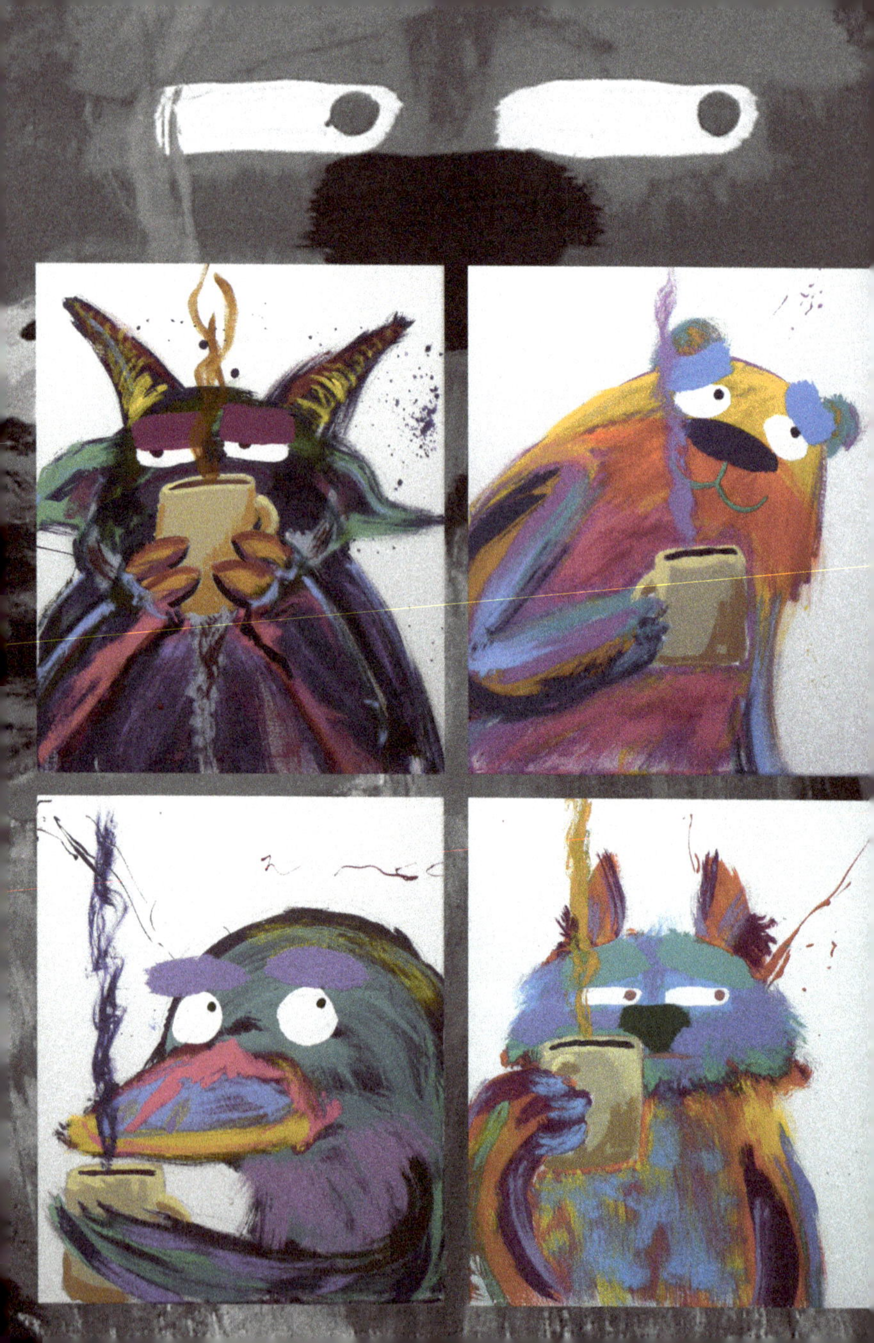

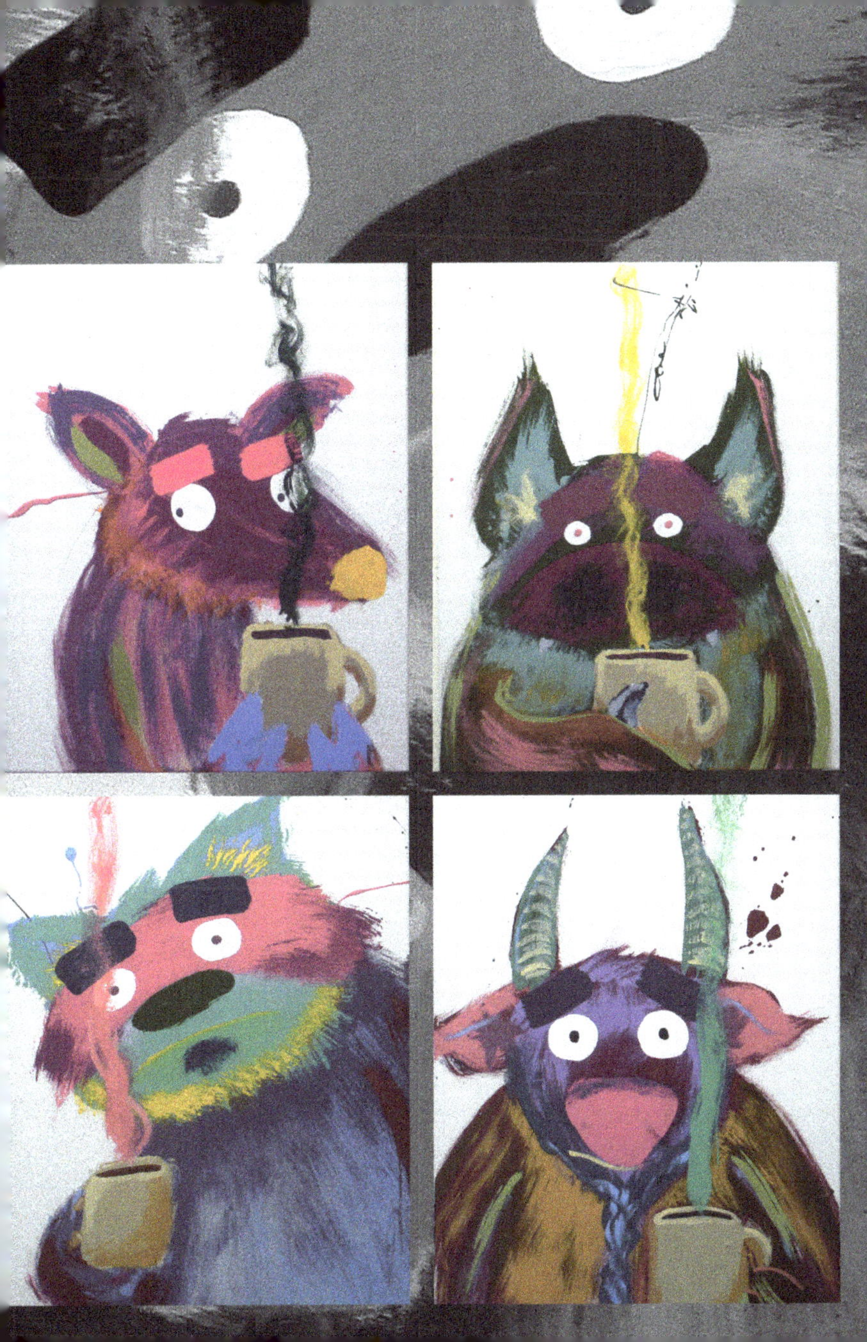

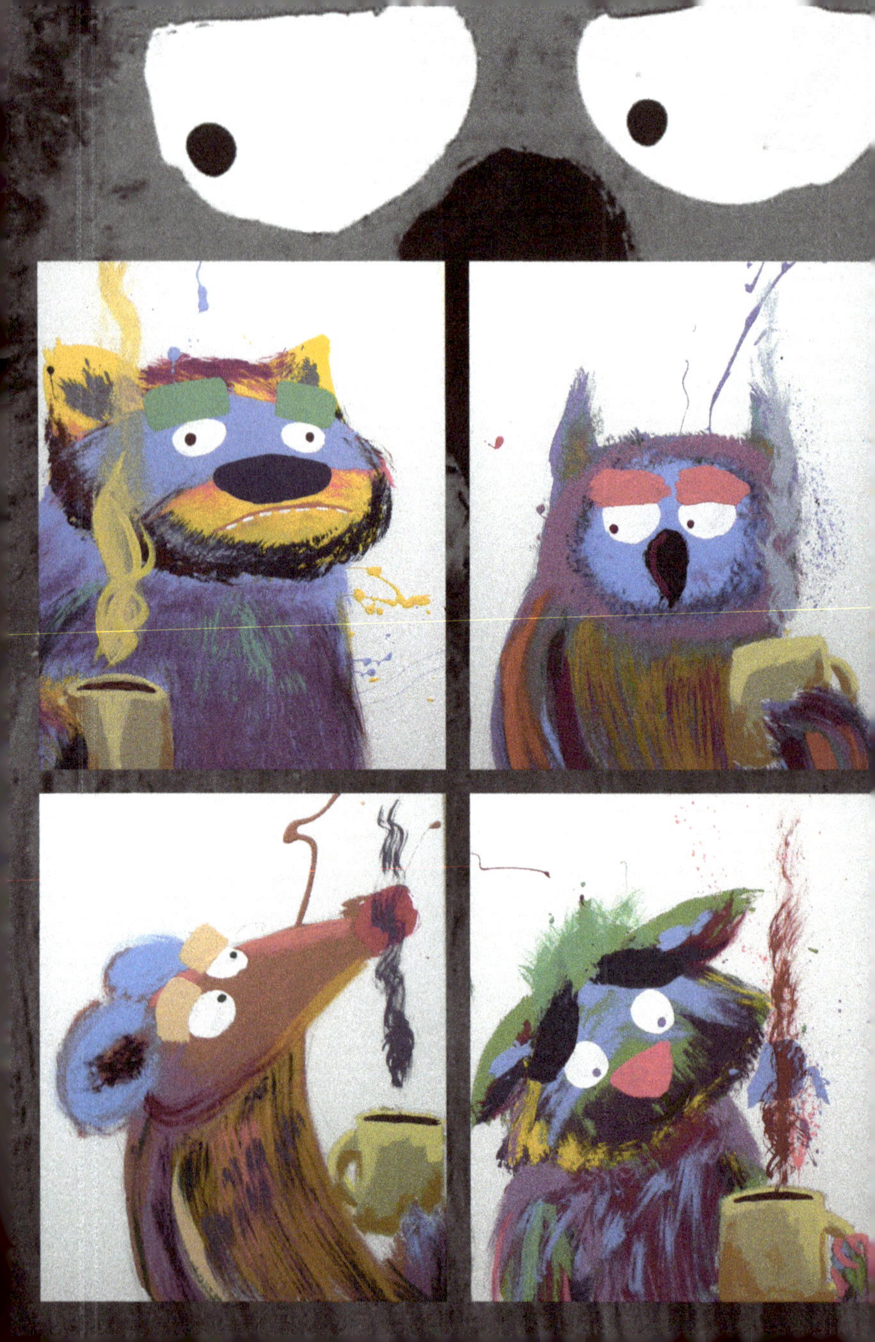

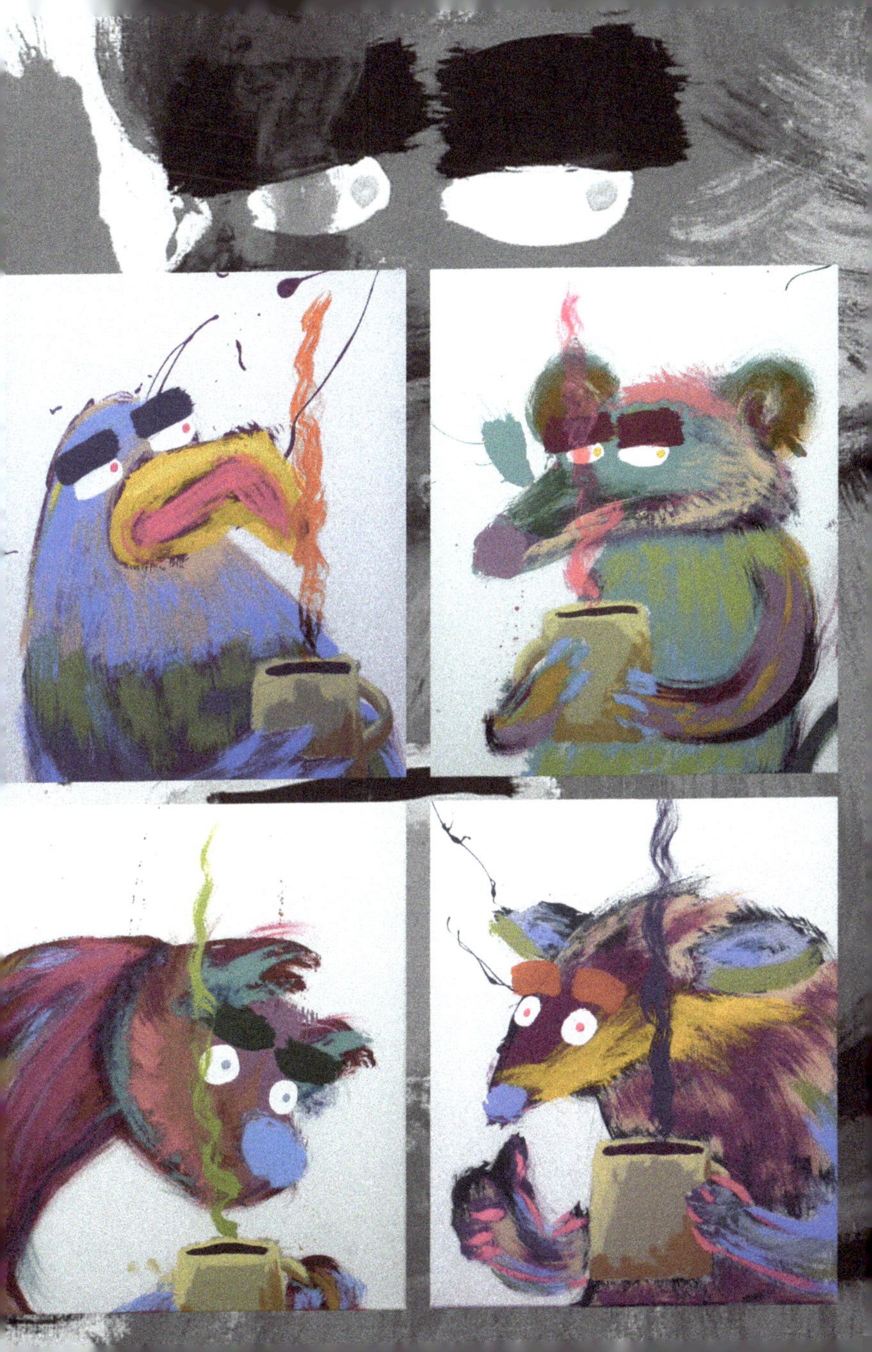

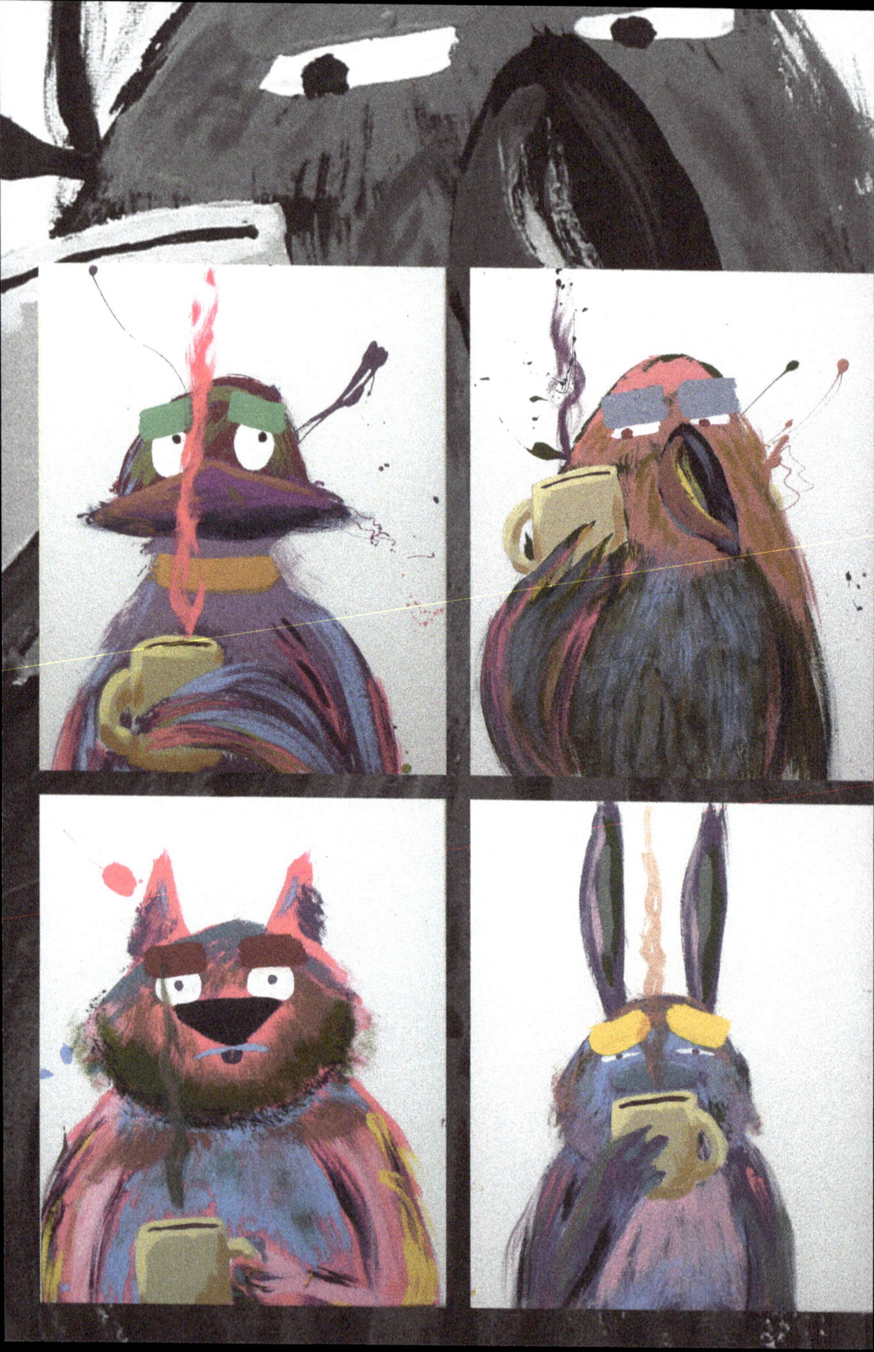

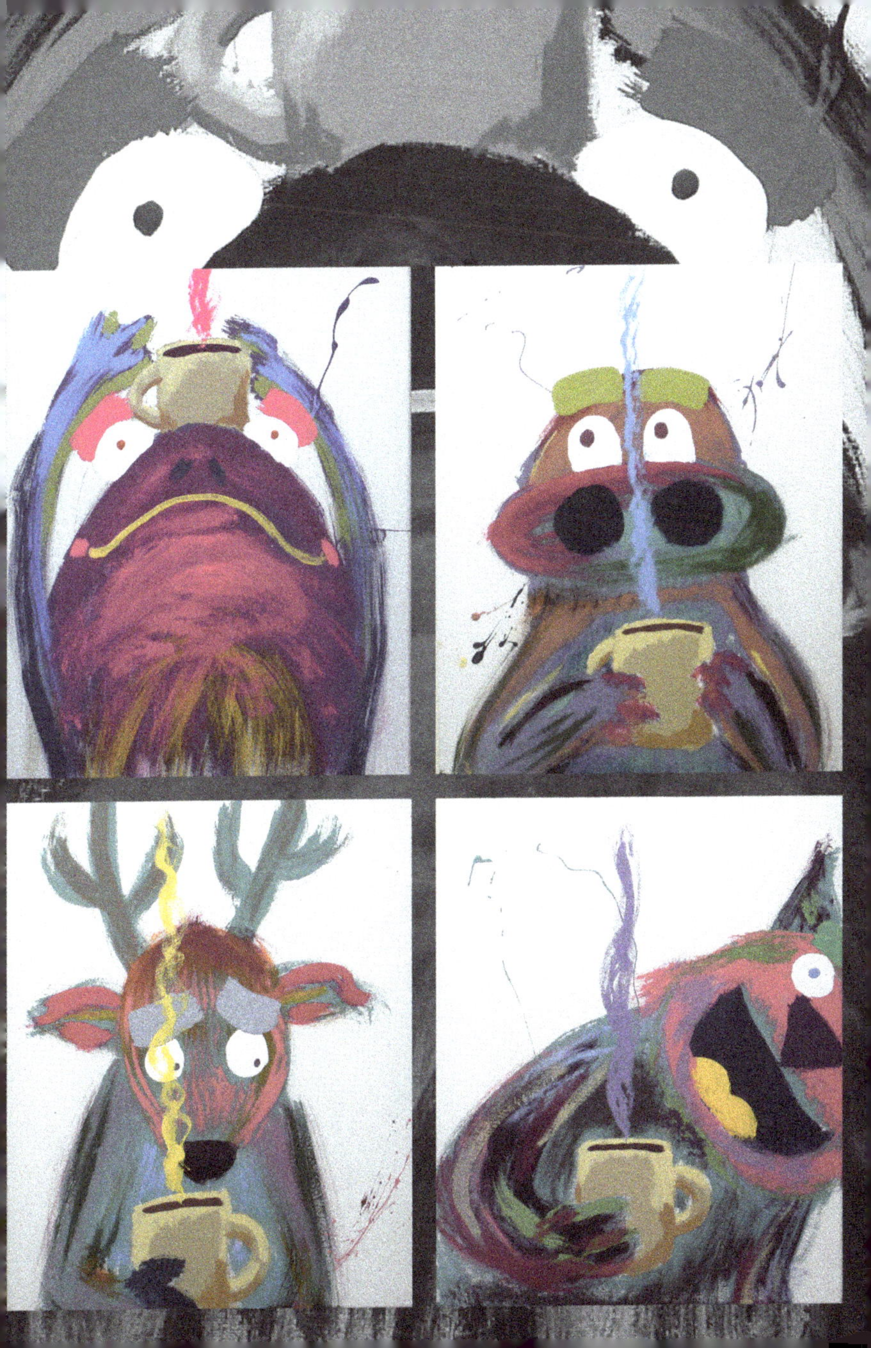

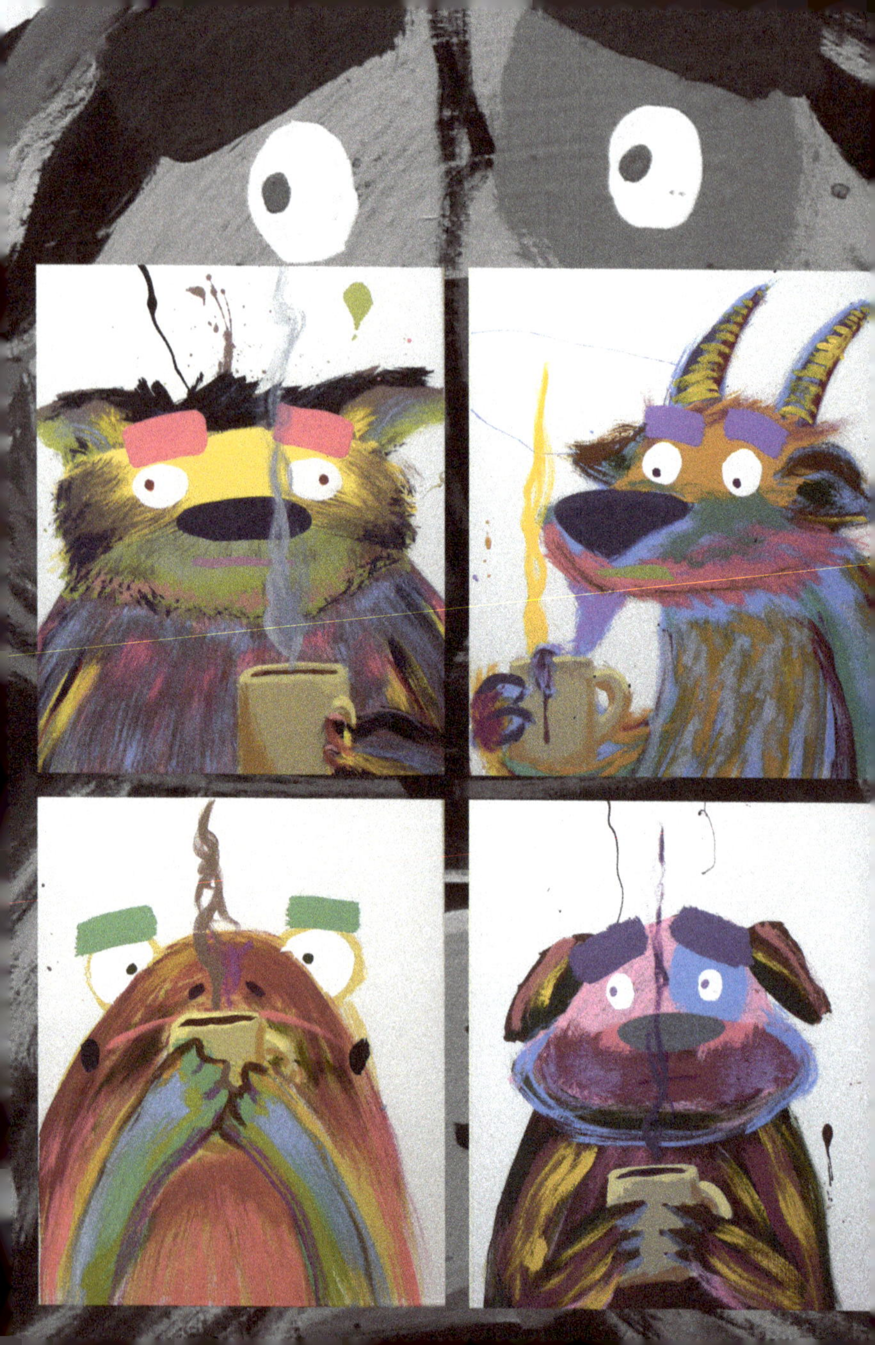

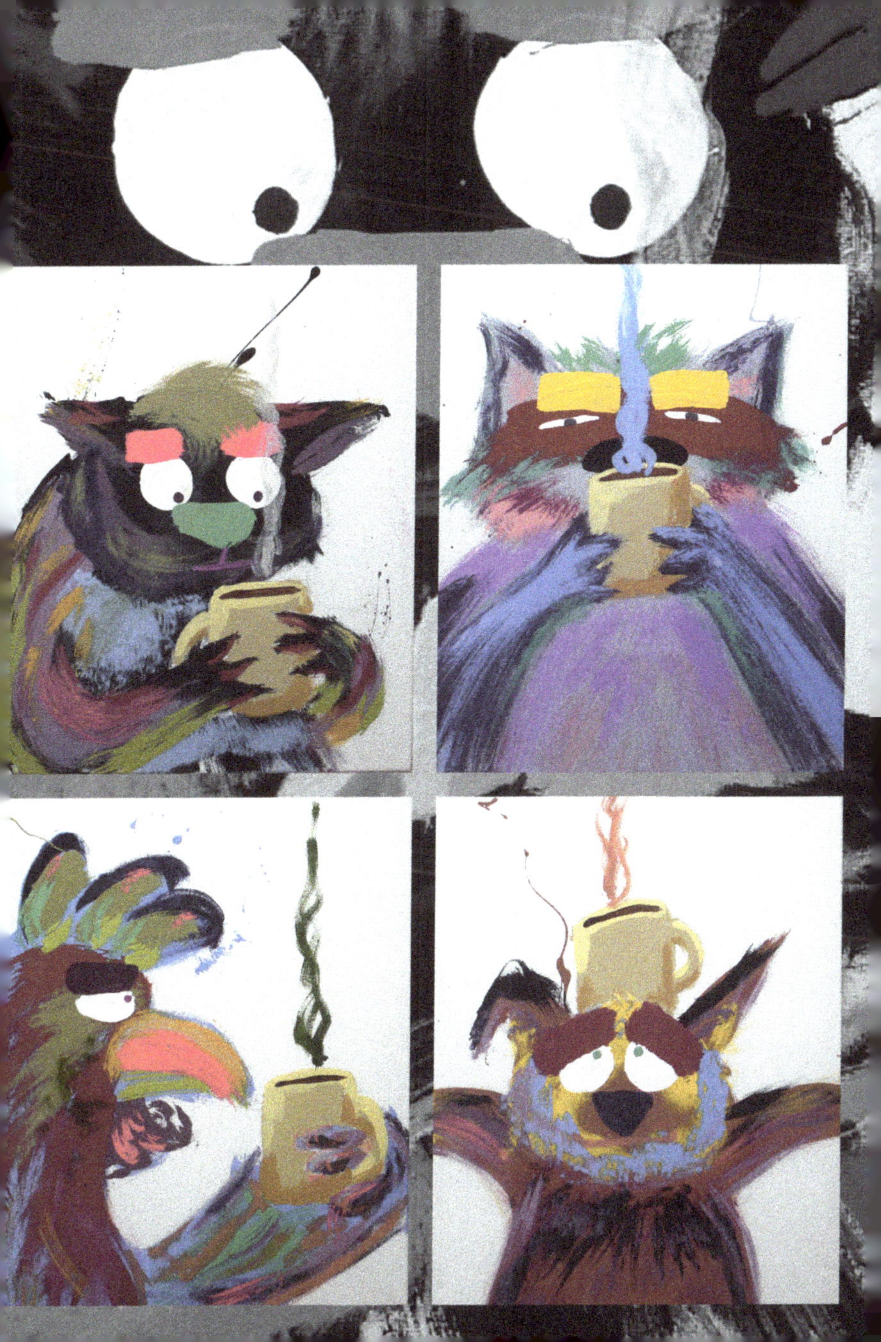

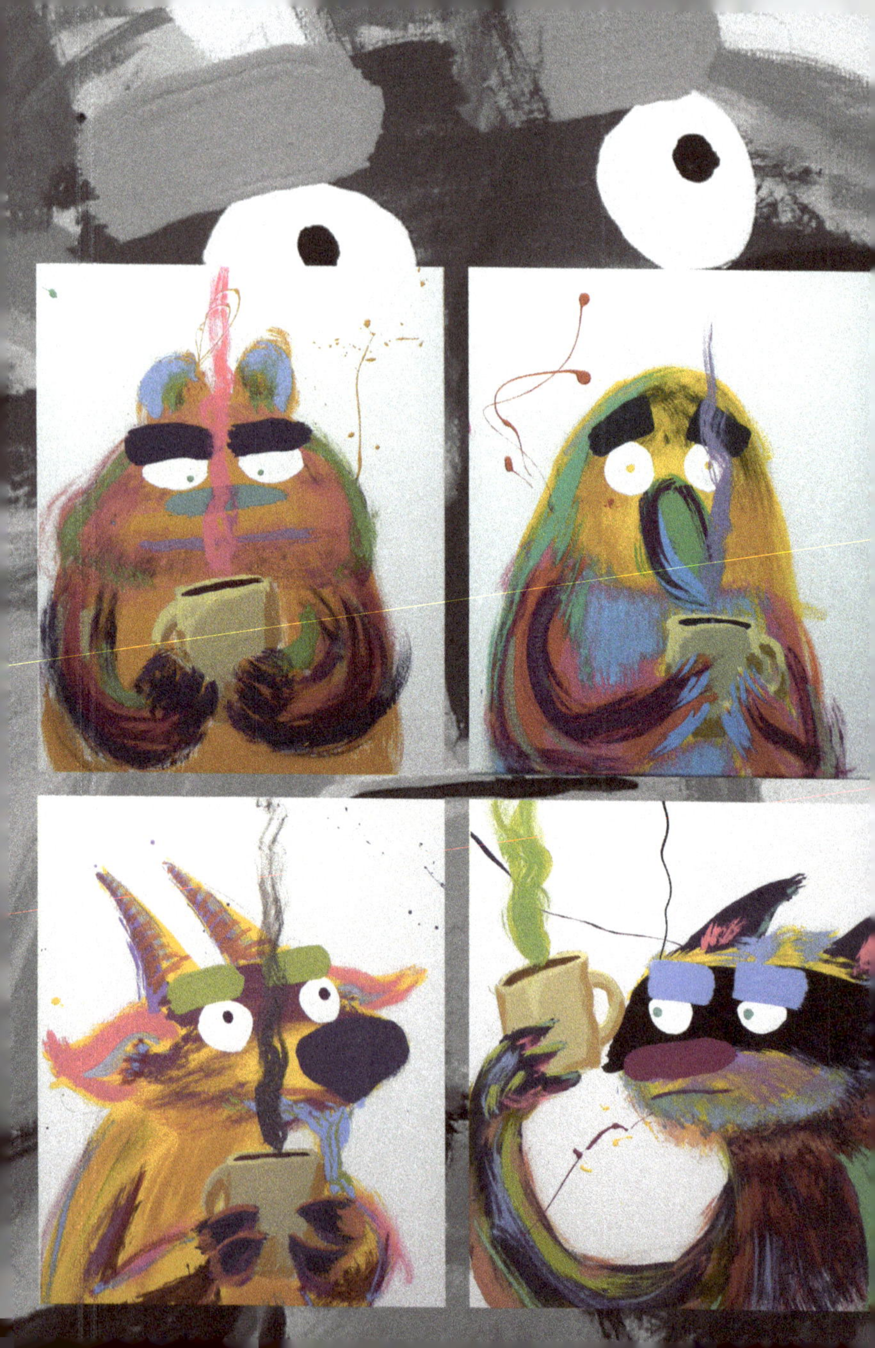

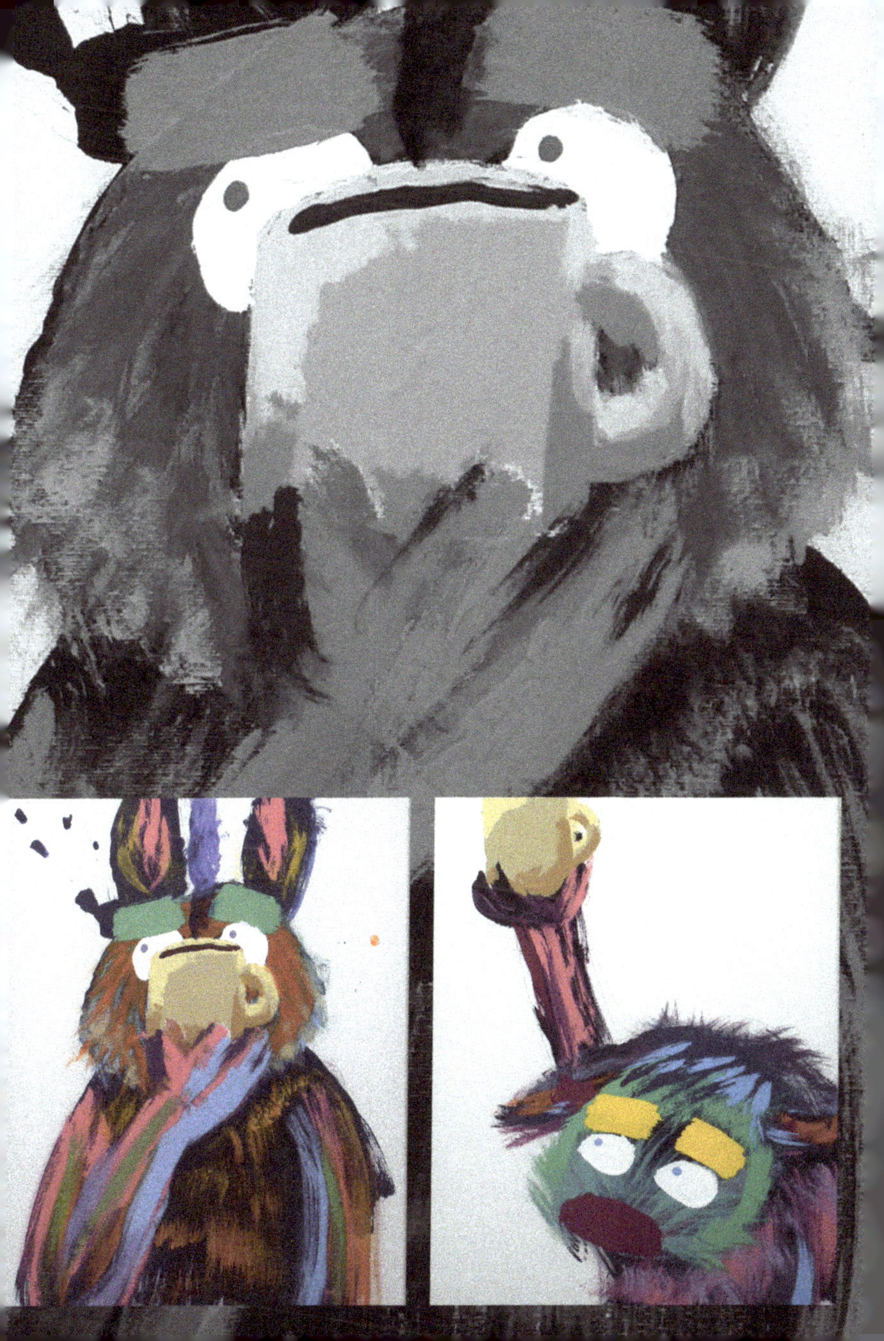

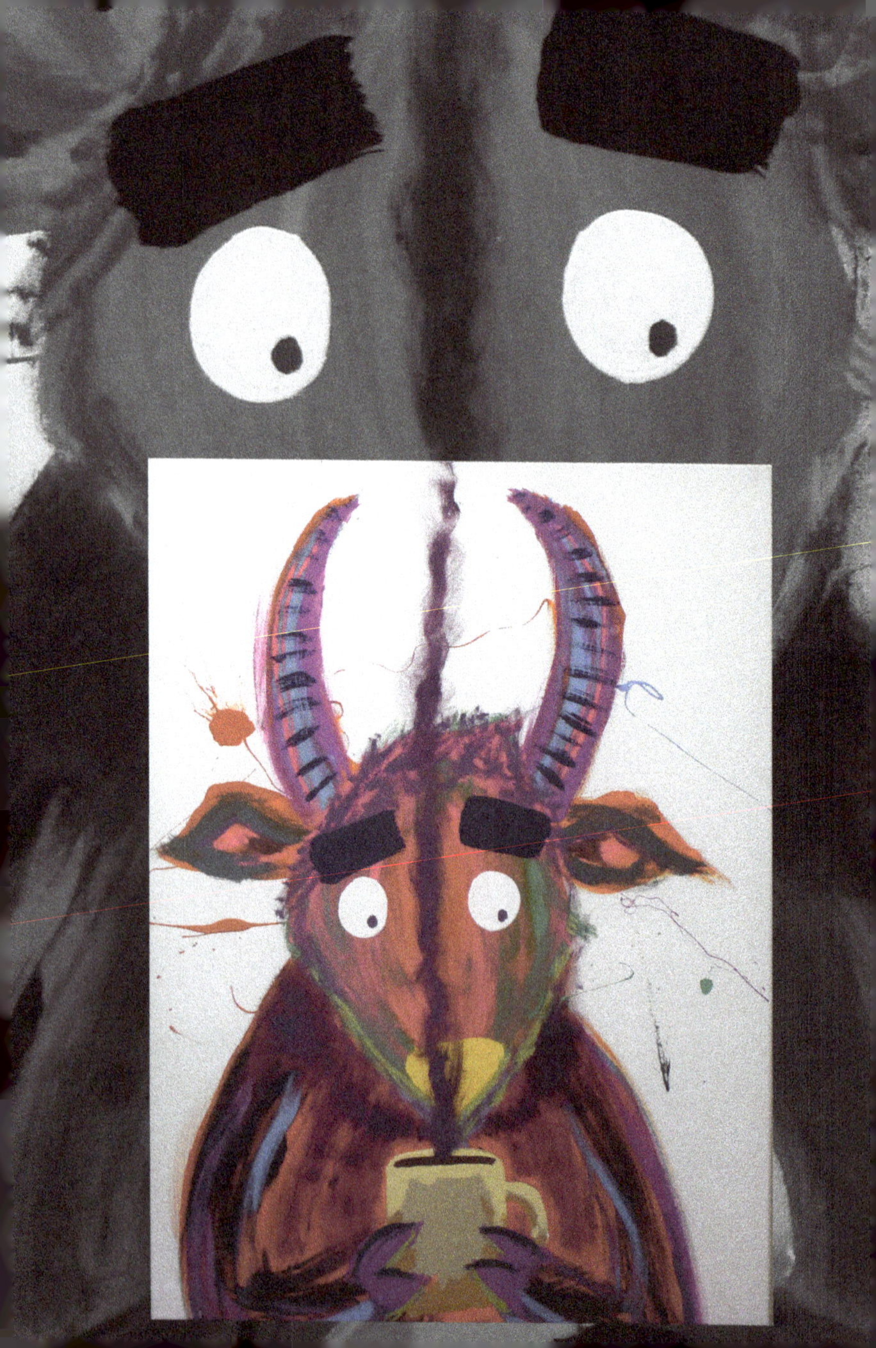

THESE PAINTINGS ARE ALL HOUSE PAINT
ON CANVAS— CREATED IN A FREEZING
COLD GARAGE, WINTER 2015.
THEY THEN FILLED THE WALLS OF THE
BATDORF & BRONSON COFFEE SHOP IN
OLYMPIA, JANUARY 2016— A TIME OF
YEAR USUALLY RESERVED FOR DARK
NEUTRAL COLORS AND SOMBER MITTENS.
ALL PAINTINGS WERE 16"x20" EXCEPT FOR
THE TWO THAT WERE BIGGER.
THE PAINTINGS WERE HUNG AT THE
SAME EXHIBITION WHERE THE BOOK
WAS PRESENTED — SO WE THOUGHT.
"HEY— WHY NOT INCLUDE THEM HERE?"
THERE YOU GO.

SPECIAL THANKS TO SIGNE
AND THE FINE PEOPLE AT
BATDORF & BRONSON FOR
HELPING MAKE THIS
SILLY PROJECT POSSIBLE.

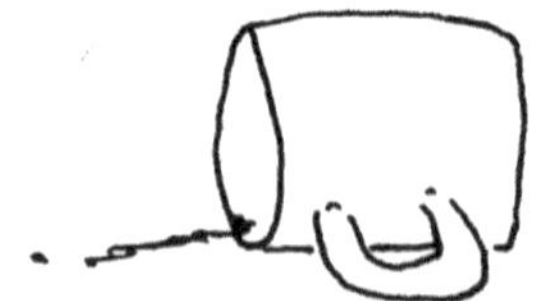